My Child Won't Eat!

My Child Won't Eat!

How to enjoy mealtimes without worry

Carlos González

My Child Won't Eat!

First published in the US by La Leche League International Ltd 2005
This second edition first published in Great Britain by Pinter & Martin Ltd 2012

© Carlos González Rodríguez, 1999
© Planeta Madrid, S.A., 1999, 2004
   Paseo de Recoletos 4, 4ª, 28001 Madrid (Spain)

Translated into English by Norma Ortiz Escobar,
additional translation of the second edition by Lorenza Garcia

ISBN 978-1-78066-005-9

Also available as an ebook

British Library Cataloguing-in-Publication Data
A catalogue record for this book is available from the British Library

Printed in Great Britain by TJ International Ltd, Padstow, Cornwall

Pinter & Martin Ltd
6 Effra Parade
London SW2 1PS

www.pinterandmartin.com

Contents

Acknowledgements

The mother's stories that are included in this book come from letters that were received by the magazine *Ser Padres* (*Being Parents*).

Names and identifying characteristics have been changed to protect the privacy of those involved. I am truly grateful to all those writers for the trust they have placed in me and for the many things they have taught me. An early version of the story "The Charge of the Nutrition Brigade" that concludes this book was published in the above magazine in February of 1998.

I would also like to thank Maite Fabregat, Joana Guerrero, Rosa Maria Jové, Margarita Otero, Cristina Ros, and Pilar Serrano for their valuable comments about the manuscript.

About the author

Carlos González, a father of three, studied medicine at the Universidad Autónoma de Barcelona and trained as a paediatrician at the Hospital de Sant Joan de Déu. The founder and president of the Catalan Breastfeeding Association (ACPAM), he currently gives courses on breastfeeding for medical professionals. Since 1996 he has been breastfeeding correspondent for *Ser Padres* (*Being Parents*) magazine. He followed the success of *My Child Won't Eat!*, with the bestselling *Kiss Me!*, published for the first time in English by Pinter & Martin.

To my mother,
who fed me while sitting
on the windowsill.

Foreword

In recent years the knowledge of appetite physiology has made remarkable advances. We marvel at the complex processes that regulate the intake of food. However, it is still amazing how many myths persist when it comes to a child's appetite, and the numerous rules that are imposed upon infant and child feeding.

My first painful experience with these rules was when I witnessed my younger brother's distress. I was about three and he must have been about two years old. That afternoon we were under the care of an aunt who was usually a kind and loving caretaker.

My brother refused to eat the banana that had been allotted to him as a snack. So she took him in her arms, pinched his nose, and when he had to open his mouth to breathe, she inserted the banana without a hint of compassion. She continued doing this in spite of his cries and struggles to get free until he finished the entire banana. I perceived this as an act of cruelty, the purpose of which I did not understand. If he were hungry, he would have eaten, and if he wasn't eating it was because he wasn't hungry! Even a three-year-old child understands this.

I could also tell some tales about the school lunchroom. Under the tables you could find almost anything: most common were slices of bread, oranges and hot dogs. Sometimes there were even whole eggs. I don't know if the principal knew it, or if she thought the children ate all their food, but I'm sure the janitor was well aware of how much a child can eat.

After many years of study, I have confirmed my first

impression. It is appetite that regulates the intake of food, and at least in children, it does so in a way that adequately meets their needs. Each animal species has food preferences that seem to be genetically determined. We are not the exception, at least before we acquire the habits of the times in which we are born. As the years go by we learn to eat according to different motivations: because it is Christmas or Easter or because we want to please our mother-in-law or look good in a bikini. Children, however, do not have preconceived ideas about how much or when to eat. Neither do they know (nor do they need to know) the doctor's recommendations, nor the recommendations from the World Health Organization, nor how much the neighbour's child eats. This is one reason they do not easily accept the rigid rules that are sometimes imposed on them.

Children do know. We should pay attention and learn, both in regard to food and in many other things. One time, before nursing my son, I asked in a loud voice (so that others in the room who were sceptical about my breastfeeding could hear): "Darling, do you want to drink some species-specific milk that has evolved over the course of millions of years until it's perfect just for you? This milk won't cause allergies and it will protect you from many illnesses." Perplexed, he looked at me and said: "Nooooo, I wan nummies!"

This book, which is easy to read and scientifically sound, as well as respectful to mothers and their children, also shines because of its underlying philosophy about the parent/child relationship. *My Child Won't Eat* will be of interest not only to those mothers who wish for a child who eats "properly," but especially to all the children who dream of enjoying mealtimes as well as all other times with their mothers.

Pilar Serrano Aguayo, MD
Endocrinology and Nutrition Specialist
Seville, Spain

Introduction

Are there any children who *do* eat?

"My child won't eat." This, or some variation of this, is one of the concerns doctors are most often confronted with. Although in winter it must compete with coughs and runny noses, "bad eaters" become the focus of questions in a doctor's surgery during the summer months.

Some mothers, like Elena, are only mildly worried:

My son, Alberto, turned one on June 20th. He is not a good eater. In fact I have to entertain him to get him to eat and even then he never cleans his plate. I don't know if I should worry, especially since he is an alert and happy child and his doctor says he is healthy.

Others, like Maribel, are close to despair:

I have an almost six-month-old who weighed 2.4 kg (5 lbs 5 oz) at birth. She is now 6.4 kg (14 lbs 1 oz) at five months. The doctor told us to start introducing food: cereal, pureed fruit, etc. However, my baby refuses to eat the food. I try every day and I am lucky if she eats a tablespoon at a time. The end result is always tears, which makes me very upset and sad. I feel bad because I don't know if I'm doing things right. I don't like to scold her and I don't want to force her to eat, but if I don't, I'm afraid she won't eat anything at all! Do you think I should wait a while before I try again? Anytime she sees a spoon she starts fussing. I feel guilty.

Would Maribel feel better if her doctor, like Elena's, told her not to worry because her daughter is healthy? "Bad eaters" become a concern because of the difference between what the child eats and what his family expects him to eat; the problem disappears when the child starts showing a heartier appetite (by eating more), or when the expectations of those around him change. It is nearly impossible (which is a good thing, since it can be dangerous) to get a child to eat more. The purpose of this book is to help the reader lower his/her expectations and align them more with reality.

You are not alone

After explaining the habits of their bad eaters, many mothers add: "I know lots of unreasonable mothers complain about the same thing, but doctor, my child really does not eat a thing. You'd have to see for yourself . . ."

They are wrong on two counts. First, they think their child is the only one who won't eat. He isn't even the one who eats the least. Certainly, dear reader, there are other children out there who eat less than yours. (And how do I know this? It's simply a matter of probability. There is in the world only one child and one alone who "eats the least of all". It's possible that his mother may not even buy this book, and even if she did, I am only likely to be wrong one time.)

But they are wrong especially to think that those other mothers are being "unreasonable". They are not. Their children really do eat very little (because they need very little as we will explain later), and their mothers are truly and genuinely worried.

Why it hurts us so much

Mothers worry, as is to be expected, about the health of their child. But there is something else that makes "bad" eating a problem that goes beyond a cough or runny nose. On the one hand, the mother tends to believe (or is made to believe) that the problem is her fault: she has not prepared the food appropriately, does not know how to feed the baby, or has not taught the child how to eat. On the other hand, mothers tend to take this personally. As Laura states:

> *My daughter is eighteen months old and she will not eat. I lovingly prepare her food only to have her spit it out after the first two teaspoons. I get so upset! What can I do to get her to eat like the good Lord intended?*

Not only is this girl a picky eater, but also to top it off she dares to "waste" her mother's efforts in the kitchen. By the way, we did not know that the "good Lord" had rules about how a child should eat. Perhaps she meant to say, "like the doctor expects"?

Many mothers express this deep personal feeling, sometimes saying: "He won't eat what I give him", or "He won't eat for me", not just, "He won't eat." Some feel this problem is a hostile act on the part of their child: "He refuses anything I offer." Many mothers have told me they shed tears at mealtimes. The poor child is sometimes involved in a false emotional conflict. Instead of raising the simple question, "Are you hungry or not?", the battle over food can become a question of "Do you love me or not?" The child is deemed guilty of not loving his mother because he simply cannot eat another bite. And not a few times the insinuation is made, sometimes even voiced directly, that "Mummy won't love you if you don't eat."

Why it hurts them more

Families, but mothers especially, become very distressed over conflict surrounding food. They truly suffer. As one of them wrote: "It's awful to be afraid of mealtimes."

If the mother is afraid, what is going on with the child? No matter how distressed you might be, please bear in mind that your child will be even more so. He is not trying to con you, manipulate you, nor is he trying to challenge you or to wilfully disobey. He is simply terrified.

I am worried about my son (fifteen months old) because he won't eat. He holds food in his mouth and spits it out after a while.
He cries the whole while and he only stops crying when I stop feeding him.

For a mother, there is always a way of escape, some comfort and hope. You may be worried because your child won't eat, fearful that he might get sick, overwhelmed because family and friends look at you and insist, "He must eat more", as if you were neglecting to feed your child. You feel rejected by a child who refuses that which is so lovingly offered and you feel guilty when you see that child cry and you sense that you might be harming him. However, it is also true that you are an adult, with all the resources of your intelligence, education and experience. You can count on the love and support of your family and friends, who most likely are on your side in this conflict. Your world, although for a time focused on child-rearing, includes more than this task. You have a certain history and a future, maybe a career. You have a certain explanation, be it true or not, about what is happening. You know why you are trying to make your child eat (even if you are baffled that he won't) and in your deepest moments of despair you keep telling yourself, "It's for his own good." You also have hope, because you know that older children eat alone and that this early stage of your feeding him will only last a couple of years.

But what about your child? What past, future, education, friends, rational explanation, or hope does he have? Your child has only you.

For a baby, his mother is his world. She is his security, his love, his warmth and his food. In her arms he is contented; when she walks away, he cries as if heartbroken. Faced with any need, any difficulty, he only has to cry and his mother answers in an instant and makes all things better.

A while ago, however, things changed. The child cries because he has eaten too much, but instead of listening as she always does, his mother tries to force him to eat even more. Things keep getting worse: her soft insistence at first soon gives way to scolding, pleading and threats. The child cannot understand the reason. He has no idea if he has eaten less than what the book said, or less than the doctor recommended, or less than the neighbour's child eats. He has not heard about calcium, iron, or vitamins. He cannot understand that you believe this is for his own good. He only knows his stomach hurts from too much food and that the food keeps coming. For him, his mother's behaviour is as baffling as if she were to smack him or leave him naked on a balcony.

Many children spend hours, sometimes up to six hours every day "eating" or, more accurately, fighting with their mothers, beside a plate of food. They don't know why. They don't know how long the battle will take (in their minds it lasts forever). No one gives them a reason; they have no one to encourage them on. The person they love the most in the world, the one whom they can usually trust, seems to have turned against them. Their whole world is crumbling.

Basic theory

Many books and magazine articles have addressed the topic of children who don't seem to want to eat. Neighbours, relatives, and friends are also quick to give advice. Their opinions don't always agree and at times even contradict each other. These differences stem in part from the answers (not always stated) that the individual advising has given to two basic questions:

1. Is the child eating enough, or should he eat more?
2. Is the child the victim or the cause of the situation?

Those who believe that "bad eaters" should eat more attribute the situation to several root causes, and accordingly propose differing solutions:

1. **Discipline.** The real fault lies with the parents who have spoiled their child, giving in to his demands and allowing him to run the show.
2. **Marketing.** The child does not eat because parents have not known how to "sell" the product. They should feed the child in a calm and relaxed environment with a beautifully decorated child's place-setting.
3. **Creative cooking.** The child is bored with the monotony in the diet. You must vary the flavours and textures while preparing attractive-looking plates: sculpt a mouse out of boiled rice with ears made out of ham, or decorate mashed potatoes with a bell pepper and olives in the shape of a clown face.
4. **Physical therapy.** You must massage the child's cheeks daily from birth, to "stimulate and strengthen" the jaw muscles.
5. **"Laissez-faire".** The child refuses food because he is showing his opposition against those who would force him to eat. If you stop making him eat, then he will eat more.

I do not agree with any of these theories. The theory that I am espousing here is similar to the one I have labelled "laissez-faire"; there is however, one fundamental difference. I do not believe that a child will eat more when you stop making him eat, because I do not believe that the child needs more food. While it is true that some children do eat more once they are not made to eat, and I have observed some who have suddenly gained weight once they are no longer forced, the weight gain is usually small: 100 or 200 g (3.5 or 7 oz) and the effect lasts only for a few days. This does not surprise me since I am convinced that not even a child's natural desire to fight against oppression can make him eat substantially less than what he needs. He may have at most a little "delayed hunger", but he will quickly make up the difference.

The idea of not forcing a child to eat is the central thesis of this book. It shouldn't be considered as a method to make your child eat more, but as a manifestation of your love and respect for him. When you stop forcing food, your child will still eat the same amount, but without the anguish and fights that up to now may have accompanied each meal.

Regarding the second question: is the child the victim or the cause of the situation? Many authors believe that a child who "won't eat" is testing the limits, showing his "strong will", obtaining a benefit and manipulating his parents. I don't agree at all. I believe that the child is the main victim in a situation that he has not caused. Read as an example the following description from Brenneman (1932), quoted by the famous English paediatrician, R. S. Illingworth, in his book *The Normal Child* (1991).[1]

> In innumerable homes there is a daily battle. On the one side the army advances with coaxing, teasing, urging, cajoling, spoofing, wheedling, begging, shaming, scolding, nagging, threatening, bribing, punishing, pointing out and demonstrating the excellence of the food, again weeping or pretending to weep, playing the fool, singing a song, or showing a picture book, turning on the radio, beating a drum just as the food enters the mouth with the hope that it will keep going in instead of returning, even having the grandmother dance a jig – all regularly recurrent actual practices encountered daily.

Up to this point, I couldn't agree more. I would continue by adding: "In the other camp the poor child defends himself as best he can: closing his mouth, spitting food out, or throwing up." However, Brenneman sees things very differently:

> On the other side a little tyrant resolutely holds the fort, either refusing to surrender, or else capitulating on his own terms. Two of his most powerful weapons of defence are vomiting and dawdling.

Why call him a tyrant? The child always suffers the most in these conflicts. Is it that some child somewhere was able to get a strawberry yogurt instead of vegetables and meat by refusing to eat? Children have many methods that are far more pleasant in order to obtain a strawberry yogurt. Do people really believe that fighting for an hour with his mother, spitting, crying, and throwing up is only a "show" in order to obtain a strawberry yogurt?

Part I
Causes

Chapter 1
How it all starts

Why do we eat?

As my mother used to say: God could have made us in such a way that we never needed to eat. As I face the daily dilemma every parent fears, "What's for dinner?", I must agree with her.

It can be a pain. Yet that is the way we are made. We must eat. Have you ever asked yourself why?

Without trying to go into philosophical complexities, we could say that eating has three primary purposes: we eat to live, to grow (or gain weight), and to move.

- **To stay alive.** Our body needs a great deal of food to simply keep functioning. Even if we spent twenty-four hours a day asleep, and even if our body had stopped growing, we would still need food.
- **To grow or gain weight.** Our muscles and bones, blood and fat, even our hair and nails are made out of what we eat.
- **To move, work and play.** We need energy to move. Everyone knows that athletes and manual labourers need to eat more than someone with an office job, and that exercise makes everyone hungry.

How much does a child need to eat?

Why do children eat?

To stay alive. The amount of food an organism needs, aside from what is needed for movement and growth, depends basically on its size. An elephant eats more than a cow and a cow eats more than a sheep. If you buy a dog, be careful when choosing the breed: a German Shepherd will eat more than a Miniature Poodle.

If children were not growing, they would need much less food than an adult, because of their smaller size.

To grow. The faster a child is growing, the more food he will need. But children are not always growing at the same rate.

What is the fastest stage of growth for a human being? It is in the womb. In nine short months, one single cell, which weighs much less than a gram, becomes a beautiful 3 kg (6 lbs) baby. Thankfully, during this time there is no need to feed the child. All the nutrients automatically go through the placenta, straight to the baby.

After birth many would say that the time of greatest growth is adolescence, the famous "teen growth spurt". But this is not true. During the teen growth spurt, growth is typically less than 10 cm (4 in) and 10 kg (22 lbs) per year. During his first year, a newborn grows 20 cm (8 in) and gains between 6 to 7 kg (13 to 15 lbs). In other words, he triples his weight; he will not triple his weight again until he is ten years old. Aside from intrauterine life, a person never grows as quickly as during the first year of life. (Bear in mind that the numbers quoted here are based on averages that have been rounded up; but each child is different and no one should become alarmed if their child is off by a few centimetres or kilos.)

It is estimated that in the first four months, babies use 27 percent of what they eat in order to grow.[2] Between six and twelve months, they only use 5 percent of what they eat to grow and in their second year, barely 3 percent. This quick growth rate is the reason babies eat so much. Due to their small size and the fact that they don't move much, they could survive with much less food if they were not growing.

Do babies eat a lot? If you don't believe they do, we can play a game. Pretend a child is not growing and that he only needs an amount of food proportional to his size. In other words, a 30 kg (66 lbs) child would eat twice as much as a 15 kg (33 lbs) child and half as much as a 60 kg (132 lbs) adult. (Of course this is not an exact proportion, so you nutritionists out there: do not get upset. In reality small animals eat more proportionally than larger animals. I am just trying to make a visual representation of the relationship between size and intake.)

According to this proportion, if a 5 kg (11 lbs) baby takes in 750 ml (25 oz) of milk in a day, then a woman weighing 50 to 60 kg (110 to 132 lbs) would have to take in ten to twelve times more, which would be 7.5 to 9 litres (2 to 2.5 gallons) of milk. Could you drink all that? Surely not. For his size, your baby eats more than you. Much more. This can be explained by the fact that he is growing and you are not.

To move. Small children move a lot, and it's common to hear phrases such as: "I don't know where he gets all his energy, with how little he eats", or "No wonder she does not gain any weight, she uses up everything she eats!"

If we stop to think about this, we also see that many children don't move much. Newborn babies move very little, and one-year-olds walk slowly and in short spurts. They get a ride everywhere they go. They don't really "work". They don't lift weights. Not even their own weight; an adult expends more energy than a child to traverse the same distance, because it takes more energy to move 60 kg (132 lbs) than it does to move 10 kg (22 lbs). "Just to look at them, it wears you out . . ." is another comment on the tireless energy of children. It may well be true, but it is unlikely that a small child uses up more energy in his playtime than a grown woman shopping for groceries.

Eating to live or living to eat?

One of the greatest myths surrounding the nutrition of young children is the idea that "you have to eat so you can grow". Many people believe growth is the consequence of good nutrition. It is not. Growth is only affected in cases of true malnutrition. If you buy a Miniature Poodle, you can feed it for a small amount of money. If you buy a German Shepherd, you may go broke buying dog food. Do you truly believe that if you feed your Miniature Poodle more, you'll end up with a German Shepherd?

The truth is children do not grow because of what they eat; they eat because they are growing. The size and bulk of a German Shepherd or a Miniature Poodle are firmly anchored in their genes; each animal ingests the amount of food (not more or less) that it needs to reach its normal size. The same is true for humans: Those who will be tall, big-boned adults will always eat more than those who will be short and thin.

The child between one and six years of age, who grows slowly, will eat proportionally less than the fast-growing six-month-old or twelve-year-old. No matter how much you feed him, it is absolutely impossible to make a two-year-old grow as fast as a six-month-old or a fifteen-year-old. The opposite is also true. Withholding food from a child will not make him grow up to be smaller, unless he is truly malnourished. We know, for example, that the size of young army recruits increased in the last few decades, which is in part due to nutritional changes. However, the difference between those who grew up in times of war and want and those who enjoyed all the prosperity of more recent years is only a few centimetres (an inch or so).

Individual adult size depends basically on genes and only in small part on nutrition. Tall parents tend to have tall children. The rate of growth in a specific timeframe depends basically on the age of the child, and only a little on genetics. A thirteen-year-old girl, no matter how short all her family is, will grow quicker than a three-year-old. And she will be hungrier.

Why they don't want vegetables

I can't get my seven-month-old daughter to eat vegetables.

I am not surprised. My eighty-nine-year-old father has never eaten cooked vegetables in his entire life (unless you consider tomato sauce a vegetable). He does eat some salad. Before he married, when he spent long work seasons in boarding homes, he would always tell the cook he had an ulcer. He would say that the doctor had forbidden him to eat vegetables. As impossible as this diet seems, he always managed to receive special meals for his "infirmity". As a result of his particular aversion, we never ate vegetables at home because my mother didn't even bother to buy them.

My father loathes vegetables more than any other person that I know. When I was preparing to write this book, I asked him his reasons. His answer was: "They tried to make me eat them. My mother would set out the vegetables and no matter how much I said I didn't care for them, she would insist all the more until I was sent to bed without any supper." He adds that not even during the war was anyone able to make him eat vegetables and that once he went without food for three whole days because all that was available were vegetables.

In the early 1900s (see the Appendix, "A bit of history", on page 166), vegetables as well as fruits were introduced very late in children's diets: perhaps at two or three years of age and with great caution. Since they were breastfed, children were fine without them because human milk provided all the necessary vitamins. When artificial feeding started becoming more widespread, babies started becoming deficient in some vitamins (due to the fact that it took manufacturers decades to add all the necessary vitamins to artificial baby milks). This made it necessary to introduce fruits and vegetables much earlier. But there was a problem: their low caloric density.

Small children have smaller stomachs. They need concentrated foods, high in calories but low in volume. This is one of the main causes of infant malnutrition. In many countries, children are malnourished but adults are not. It would be a mistake to believe that adults eat everything and leave nothing for the children. Parents (and especially mothers) both here and anywhere else watch out for their children. They would happily give up their own food in order to feed their children. The problem is that many times the only food available to families consists of vegetables and roots high in fibre but low in calories. Adults can eat all they need, as their stomachs are big enough. And in enough quantity, any food will fatten a person. Small children, as hard as they try, cannot eat the amount of vegetables needed, because they don't have enough room in their stomach.

Mother's milk has 70 kcal (kilocalories, commonly known as calories) per 100 g (3.5 oz). By contrast boiled rice has 126 kcal, cooked chickpeas (garbanzos) 150 kcal, chicken 186 kcal, bananas 91 kcal per 100 g (3.5 oz) – but apples have only 52 kcal, oranges 45 kcal, cooked carrots 27 kcal, cooked cabbage 15 kcal, cooked spinach 20 kcal, green beans 15 kcal and lettuce 17 kcal per 100 g (3.5 oz). And this is providing that these foods have been drained well; if the water they've been cooked in is included, they are even less "substantial".

A few years ago, a scientist was curious enough to analyse baby food prepared by several mothers for their children in Madrid.[3] The food was made with vegetables and meat. He discovered that the average caloric concentration was 50 kcal per 100 g (3.5 oz). This was an average. Some only had 30 kcal per 100 g. And this was with meat included. You can imagine what vegetables alone might be. Are you still wondering why your child prefers breastfeeding to vegetables? Do you still believe, "You should be feeding him more solids, otherwise, he'll never grow"?

If left alone, small children seldom refuse vegetables. It is not a matter of taste. Usually they will gladly accept a few bites of vegetables, rich in important minerals and vitamins. But only a few bites. Some mothers try to give them a plateful of these "healthy" foods. And, adding insult to injury, they aim to give them this plate of vegetables instead of the breast or bottle that often has three times the calories! "They want to starve me!" thinks the child. He is amazed at our efforts and, as is to be expected, refuses to accept such a raw deal. So the fighting begins and the child can become so adverse to fruit and vegetables that later on, when he grows and can now take them in, he no longer wants them.

Many stop eating at one year

As we have seen, babies eat much more than adults, relative to their size. This means that somewhere along the road to adulthood, they must start eating less. And usually this happens sooner rather than later, much to the surprise and horror of many mothers. Children "stop eating" approximately around twelve months of age. Some stop eating at nine months, others hold out until eighteen months or two years. A very few keep on eating, while some "have never eaten well since they were born".

The reason behind this change is the slower growth rate that we have already discussed. In the first year, babies grow more quickly than at any other time in their life outside the womb. During the second year, by contrast, the growth rate is much slower: only around 9 cm (3.5 in) and 2 kg (4.4 lbs). What ends up happening is that the energy necessary to move increases since the child moves more; the energy necessary to stay alive also increases because the child is bigger. However, the energy needed for growth diminishes enormously, resulting in a child who needs either the same amount of food or less than before. According to experts, eighteen-month-old babies eat little more than nine-month-olds; this is on average. In reality, many eighteen-month-olds eat less than they did at nine months. Parents, ignorant of this fact, make an honest mistake, thinking: "If at a year he eats this much, at two years he should eat twice as much." The result is a mother trying to feed twice as much food to a child who needs only half as much. The conflict is inevitable and violent at times.

Moreover, many babies eat very watery foods like pureed fruit and vegetables. When they are finally given solid foods, such as pasta, chicken, chips, bread or chickpeas, of course they need far smaller amounts.

How long does this phase last? The situation seems to be temporary. Upon hearing advice from grandmothers, neighbours and doctors, mothers sometimes trust that their child will "grow out of this". In fact, many children around five to seven years of age do start eating more as their size increases. But this small increase in intake is not always enough to appease the expectations of their families. On the one hand, the amount of food that any person needs varies greatly and some children eat much more or much less than their peers of the same age and size. On the other hand, parents' expectations can also vary greatly. Some mothers would be happy if the child finished the serving of macaroni, while others also want the child to eat the meat and potatoes, plus a banana and a yogurt. For some reason or another, many children remain small eaters until puberty. Then, when the slower growth of middle childhood gives way to the adolescent growth spurt, these children feel insatiable hunger and, to their mother's astonishment and joy, they eat everything in the refrigerator, "eating the family out of house and home".

One mother, Cristina, remembers clearly the moment her son stopped eating at fifteen months:

My sixteen-month-old son has always been a good eater: pureed vegetables and chicken, fish or egg, fruit, rice, pasta. The one thing he has never really liked is baby cereal. He also insists on feeding himself and we let him (even if by doing so he eats less). Our problem started about a month ago. Now he won't eat! It's not like he refuses one thing and then accepts something else. What happens is that he eats two or three bites and then he does not want any more. We have tried everything: vegetables, different consistencies, entertaining him with things (his grandparents even take him out on the balcony to feed him).

Notice what Cristina says, as if in passing: Her child "insists" on feeding himself, but that means he eats less. Between six months and one year, children often go through a phase where they want to feed themselves and enjoy doing it. Of course, they eat less, take longer, and get messy. If the mother is willing to accept these small inconveniences, her child will probably continue feeding himself for the rest of his life. If in the interest of haste and ease (and especially to make him eat more) the mother decides to feed the baby herself, it is likely that she will regret the decision a couple of years later. Two- and three-year-old children do not often show the same spontaneous interest in feeding themselves that they did when they were under one.

Others have never eaten well in their life

In some cases, "fussy eaters" start much earlier, in the early months or weeks. All humans are different and some children need much less to eat than others. Sometimes, the child is eating as much as his peers, but the mother is unaware:

> *Problems started in the hospital; each time I tried to nurse him, he would start to cry. After much insistence he would latch on for a moment and then let go. This happened every two or three hours. Once we got home, things got worse. The baby cried all day and all day long I tried to put the breast into his mouth. He seemed not to know how to nurse. My older son was also in tears since I had no time for him. Finally at three weeks I couldn't stand it anymore, so I started bottle-feeding. At first things improved, but right now things are unbearable again. Just to get him to take 100 or 120 ml (3.5 or 4.2 oz) can take up to an hour or more. Some feedings he barely takes 70 ml (2.5 oz). The only time he feeds well is after his bath when he takes 180 ml (6 oz). He only takes between 600 to 700 ml (21 to 24 oz) in twenty-four hours. He is also slow to gain weight. Some weeks he has gained less than 100 g (3.5 oz). At three months he weighs 5.800 kg (12 lbs 12 oz).*

Angela's baby's weight is totally normal, at percentile 20 (one in six children weigh less, see pages 33–5). His intake of 700 ml (24 oz) of milk (about 490 kcal), is normal, although probably less than what the doctor has recommended. Many books recommend

105 to 110 kcal per 1 kg (2.2 lbs) of weight (about 900 ml or 30 oz of milk for Angela's baby) but more recent research[4] indicates that average needs are about 88.3 kcal/kg, and the minimum need at two standard deviations is 59.7 kcal/kg, which for this baby would be 732 ml (25 oz) and 495 ml (16.7 oz) of milk. Restating this for those who got lost in the numbers, half of the three-month-old children that are bottle-fed need less than 730 ml (25 oz) and some only take 500 ml (17 oz). However, many texts still recommend 900 ml (30 oz) and some even round up to 1000 ml (35 oz). These numbers are net needs; reality shows us that children sometimes take a little more and spit up part of a feeding. Out of 380 healthy three-month-old male babies studied by Fomon,[2] 5 percent took in less than 660 ml (22 oz); and this is actual intake.

Those who are "barely on the chart"

In some cases, the problem presented is not that the nursing sessions are thought "too short", but that the child's weight gain is deemed "too little". There are people of different sizes in the world, and any morning while running errands we may come across people who weigh 50 kg (110 lbs) and others who weigh 100 kg (220 lbs). Do people really think that they all weighed the same when they were three months old? Why, then, is it so hard to accept differing weights in our children?

> I have a three-month-old baby girl whom I breastfeed. Up till now she was gaining well, 200 or 250 g (7 to 9 oz) per week. Two weeks ago I took her to the doctor and she had only gained 80 g (3 oz). She was born at 3.2 kg (7 lbs) and at her doctor's visit was 5.820 kg (12 lbs 13 oz). The doctor suggested supplementing, but when I give her the bottle, she refuses to take it. I have tried different types of formulas and nipples and she still rejects the bottle. She cries and refuses even the breast for four or five hours. I've tried to give her formula mixed in with a little cereal and to feed it with a spoon and she still

won't take it. She only wants to breastfeed. I can't go on like this; I am afraid for the health of my child, seeing that she's not gaining what she should. The doctor says she's crossed the red line.

Which red line? According to the World Health Organization (WHO) growth charts, this baby's weight is above the mean. She could weigh between 4.6 and 7.4 kg (10 lbs 2 oz and 16 lbs 5 oz). She has gained 2.620 kg (5 lbs 13 oz) in three months, more than 850 g (1 lb 14 oz) per month. The only red line that has been crossed is the one that measures this mother's endurance. How many more hours of anguish, how many trips to the store to buy new nipples and new formula will be needed, just because someone misread a chart? How many bottles does a baby have to refuse to show she doesn't want more food?

This example illustrates two fundamental problems: on the one hand, the general interpretation of weight charts; on the other, the growth rate of breastfed babies.

What are weight charts and what purpose do they serve?

On the next page is an example of a weight chart. It is totally made up so don't go looking for your child on this chart! I've simply included it to explain what each line means. There are different weight charts: United States (US) charts (which the World Health Organization used to recommend for use the world over, prior to having their own charts) and other countries' charts: France, Great Britain, Spain, etc. By the way, they do not match, and should a doctor or nurse happen to see all of them together, a whole Sunday afternoon could be spent comparing the different charts.

The numbers on the right side are called "percentiles". The 75th percentile means that out of 100 healthy children, 75 are under this line and 25 are above it. In some charts, the extreme curves are at 95 and 5, not at 97 and 3.

Other charts do not use percentiles; they use mean and standard deviations. Such charts have, from bottom to top, five lines that correspond to –2, –1, mean, +1 and +2 standard deviations. By the way, 16 percent of healthy children will be beneath the "minus one" while a little more than 2 percent will be beneath the "minus two".

We have placed on our graph the weights of three imaginary girls of the same age. Adela has totally normal weight, however only 6 percent of girls her age will weigh more. Although Ester weighs 1.5 kg (3 lbs 3 oz) less than Adela, she also has normal weight; however, 85 percent of girls her age will weigh more than her. There is no way that you can say that Ester is not doing well, has low weight, or is "barely on the chart". It is a common mistake to want all children to be above the mean. Half of all children, by definition, will be below the 50th percentile.

What about Laura? She is under the last curve, and many times this is seen as "not doing well" weight-wise. But notice: the last line is the 3rd percentile; which means that 3 percent of healthy children will be beneath this line. This is not the curve that separates the healthy children from the sick. It is only one sign that tells the doctor: "Look out for this child, although she's probably healthy, she may also be sick." So how is a doctor supposed to know which of the children who fall under the 3 percent curve are sick and which are healthy? Well, that's why the

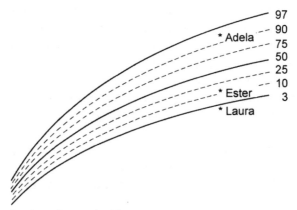

Weight chart (example A)

doctor went to medical school.

We have insisted several times that 25 percent of *healthy* children will be under the 25th percentile. The way charts are developed is by weighing hundreds or thousands of healthy children. When developing the chart, if a child is born premature, has Down's syndrome, a severe heart condition, or has spent several weeks in hospital due to severe diarrhoea, then you won't use his weight to estimate the mean for a normal weight chart. By the same token, if your child has one of these issues, his weight will probably not follow normal growth curves. A child with a chronic illness (or who has recently had an acute bout of illness) and who has been labelled "low weight" is not this way because he didn't eat, but because he's been sick. To force him to eat is not going to cure him; it will only torture him and make him throw up.

In the weight chart below (example B), we have now added two other imaginary girls to our imaginary weight chart on the previous page (example A). The one on top is Tamara; her weight, as you can see, stays between the 90th and 97th percentile. Some would say that she's "following the curve".

The lower line shows Marta's weight. We see that at one point she reaches over the 50th percentile, but later on she approaches the 10th percentile. What's up with Marta? Probably nothing. Of course, if the curve were to change too rapidly or too steeply, her

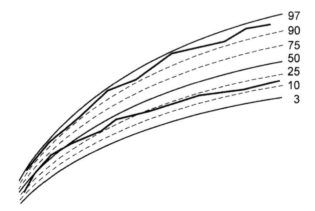

Weight chart (example B)

doctor would do well to check her to make sure that there is no underlying problem. But most likely he will find nothing wrong. Very simply, weight charts are not road maps to be followed, but more accurately, they are mathematical representations of complex statistical functions. The percentile curves do not correspond to the weight gain of one particular child, and the weight of one individual child does not have to follow any of these lines. The chart below (example C) illustrates this better.

With the sole purpose of making ourselves a place in the history of paediatrics, instead of copying United States or Spanish charts, we have devised our own charts (the first virtual charts, since we've only weighed imaginary babies). We have followed two girls and their weight through their first year. The two thick lines represent them.

The thin line is the mean of both these girls' weight. One of these girls started above the mean and then dipped below it; the other started below it and then rose above it. Neither of these girls follows the mean. Should we say that both these girls have nutrition concerns because they do not follow "the curve"? Of course not. It's the mean that does not follow these girls' "curve."

Of course, weight charts are not developed using only two girls, but several hundred. Can you imagine how complicated things can get?

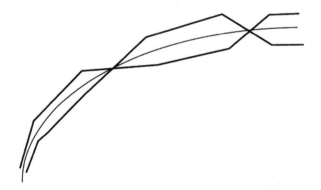

Weight chart (example C)

Growth in the breastfed baby

Marta's weight gain that we saw on page 35 is quite typical of breastfed babies. The most commonly used weight charts were developed years ago, when the majority of babies were bottle-fed, and the ones that did breastfeed, only did so for a few weeks. These days, more and more children are being breastfed in terms of months, and they do not follow the old charts. In the 1990s several studies[5,6] done in the United States, Canada, and Europe have shown that breastfed babies often gain weight much quicker in the first month than the growth charts show, but then they start slowing down and losing percentile points. By six months they have lost the head start that they had gained in the first month, and by the time they are one year old they seem to have "low" weight according to the charts.

As a result of these discoveries, the WHO produced a new series of child-growth standards based on data from children of different races who are breastfed for more than a year. After some delay, the new growth standards were finally published in 2006; you can find them at www.who.int/childgrowth/en/. There are no separate growth standards for children who are breastfed and children who are bottle-fed; the same standards apply to all.[7]

Compared to the old American child-growth standards, the new WHO ones show higher levels of growth at two or three months, but lower ones at six months and older. It seems the difference in the first few months is due to the American child-growth standards having been badly constructed, using very few data.

In Spain, the most commonly used child growth standards are those of La Fundación Orbegozo in Bilbao. During the first few months, they are virtually identical to those of the WHO both in weight and height. However, in children of five to six months or older, while height continues to be more or less the same, there is a variation in weight: the WHO child-growth standards are 300 to 500 g less. All the coordinates are lower: the 3rd percentile, the median and the 97th percentile. That is to say, while the baby in the WHO child-growth standards remains in the same percentile, the baby in the Spanish child growth standards appears to drop in percentile.

Many countries have officially adopted the WHO child-growth standards, and Spain will most likely do so in the near future. Until then, many mothers will probably be told, when their child is eight or nine months of age, that his "percentile is dropping".

Why is the growth of a breastfed baby so different from that of their bottle-fed peers? We are not quite sure, but in any case, it is not because of inadequate food intake. During the first month, when all they drink is milk, breastfed babies weigh the same or more. Between six and twelve months of age, when solids are part of their diet as well as milk, breastfed babies weigh a bit less. If the adage "human milk is no longer enough" were true (which is total foolishness since human milk always nourishes better than formula and also better than solids), then the child would be hungry and would eat more, therefore gaining the same as the bottle-fed infant. But they don't want more solids either. The difference is profound; for some reason, artificial feeding produces a rate of growth that does not match the pattern of breastfed babies.

In the first edition of this book I wrote: "We do not know the long term consequences that this excessive growth may have." Now we know. Several studies[8,9] have found that children who were breastfed less than six months have higher rates of obesity and are more likely to be overweight at four and six years of age.

Not all children grow at the same rate

I have an eight-month-old daughter and for the last four months she has not gained weight. She's the same 7.450 kg (16 lbs 6.7 oz) she was at four months and her length has only increased a little to the 71 cm (28 in) she is now. Her doctor has told me that if she does not gain this month he will order blood tests to see if she's lacking anything; if nothing shows up, then she is just not hungry and that's that . . .

She eats very little. She refuses the spoon and when I've made her eat, she has thrown up. I use a bottle for all her food: fruit, strained baby foods, and cereal.

It is certainly not "normal" (in the sense of "common") for children not to gain weight at all between four and eight months. To find out if this is not only an odd occurrence but also a sign of illness, you would need more information, including the results of the blood test that the doctor has prudently ordered to make sure this baby is not sick. But if no illness is detected, it is better to wait patiently; she's simply not hungry and that's that. Especially since it's also not too common to weigh that much at four months; she was practically in the 95th percentile. Her height at eight months is high, well above the mean.

All the blood tests came back normal and, at thirteen months, this girl weighed 8 kg (17 lbs 10 oz) and was still uninterested in food. It would seem that, instead of maintaining a slow and steady weight gain, this child gained all her weight in the first few months and then simply stopped gaining.

There is a special growth rate that often drives parents crazy. It is called "constitutional growth delay". It is only a variation of the normal, not an illness. These are children who do not follow any chart; they have their own growth curve. They are born of normal weight and may grow normally for a few months. But somewhere around the third to sixth month they hit the brakes and start growing very slowly, both in weight and length. They often "fall off the chart", going below the 3rd percentile in height and weight. Their weight, however, is adequate for their height. If the doctor orders lab work, everything is normal. For years they are on or outside the margins of the child-growth standards, and then between two and three years of age they begin to grow at a normal rate and remain close to the 3rd percentile. They usually reach puberty a little later than other children and therefore have more time to grow. They subsequently reach a completely normal size, and as adults are of average height. This is an inherited characteristic and it can be very reassuring when a grandmother remembers that the parent or an uncle "was also very small at first and never wanted to eat; the doctor was always giving him vitamins", but at the end of it all he grew. Let's see a typical example:

My daughter is eighteen months old and I am still breastfeeding her in spite of the negative comments from 99 percent of the people around me. The problem is that since she turned four months, when I returned to work, she has not eaten well. She started losing weight and right now is 73.2 cm (29 in) long and weighs 8.690 kg (19 lbs 2 oz). She's had lab work done and everything came back normal.

At eighteen months, the 3rd percentile (according to the WHO child-growth standards) is 8200g (18 lbs 1 oz) and 75 cm (30 in). However, for this girl to be 73 cm (29 in) and 8.690 kg (19 lbs 2 oz) means her weight for length is higher than the 25th percentile. This child had an appointment with an endocrinologist in order to check her level of growth hormone and her levels were normal. So all that is left is to wait a few years.

It follows that a child who is growing this slowly will eat even less than other children.

"Ever since he came down with that virus, he stopped eating"

In general terms, hunger in children will diminish gradually, but it is not uncommon for an outside event (illness, starting day care, the birth of a sibling, etc.) to trigger diminished appetite:

My baby just turned eleven months. Since we started solids he was eating beautifully until about two weeks ago. He would eat fish, chicken, or lamb . . . yet all of a sudden he's changed: now he only occasionally accepts these foods and never more than five or six bites at a time (if I try to make him eat more, he throws up). Some days I manage to give him his puree in two feedings. I don't know if this is because he's been sick for the past two weeks with a bad runny nose, fever, and cough . . .

Children, just like adults, lose their appetite when they are sick. Who hasn't been down with a bad cold and found he has no taste for food? Who hasn't had such a bad headache that he prefers to go to bed without dinner? Who hasn't had an upset stomach that prevents him from eating? This is a temporary loss of appetite; usually it lasts a few days, while the virus lasts, and then it goes away. If the child has lost weight, he might want to "catch up" for a few days by eating more than he normally does, until he recovers what he lost.

If the illness is more serious, this lack of appetite could last for weeks. The child may not regain his appetite until he has fully recovered.

When you try to make a sick child eat, the most likely outcome is that he will throw up. He may even grow fearful of eating and of the spoon, a fear that may stay, even after he's feeling better. If the child is truly hungry, you can't make him lose his appetite, even if you try to feed him by force. But if he was close to a year, an age when most children seem to lose their appetite anyway, it is likely that the illness coupled with the attempts at making the child eat may trigger the inevitable catastrophe. The child would have "stopped eating" anyway, but the conflict begins a few weeks earlier:

Ever since he had bronchitis he stopped eating. Each day he ate less. He is almost seven months old and he still will not eat.

What is worse is that the mother sometimes blames the lost appetite on the illness and, until the child starts eating, she will continue to believe (sometimes unconsciously) that he has never "fully recovered" from that virus, diarrhoea, ear infection, or strep throat. Frequently this leads the mother to insist even more vehemently that the child must eat, since she believes "he must eat in order to get better". Annabel's story shows us how extreme these vicious circles can get:

I have a sixteen-month-old little boy. Since he was nine months old he has refused to open his mouth to eat. During the summer he had diarrhoea several times and the doctor prescribed a medicine that had to be given with a spoon. Since then he has hated the spoon; at least that's what I think. The thing is that in order to get him to eat now I have to really distract him. While he is looking away, I stick in the spoon and he swallows. Sometimes, when I sneak the spoon into his mouth, he gags. But now I have a bigger problem because he clenches his teeth and I can't even get the spoon close to his mouth. Mealtimes are torture for both of us.

Too much of a good thing

What would happen to a child who really didn't eat? He would lose weight. A newborn, as mothers well know, can easily lose 200 g (7 oz) in the first two or three days, but this is soon regained if he is breastfeeding well. Let's suppose that the weight loss is much less – let's say a child loses 10 g (0.4 oz) per day. In 365 days, that would be around 3.650 kg (8 lbs). What would be left of a newborn if we were to remove 3.650 kg? Little more than an empty diaper. At the same rate of weight loss, a bigger child, weighing 10 kg (22 lbs) would disappear before our very eyes in less than three years.

What would happen if the child ate all that the adults wanted to feed him? Let's pretend that the child has eaten all he needs, and after much effort, you are able to get him to eat a bit more, let's say, enough to gain 10 g (0.4 oz) per day (over and above what he would need to gain normally). That would be around 3.650 kg (8 lbs) extra per year. At two years, instead of weighing 12 kg (26 lbs), he would weigh 19 kg (42 lbs). By ten years old, instead of weighing 30 kg (66 lbs), he would be 65 kg (143 lbs), and by age twenty, instead of 60 kg (132 lbs) his weight would be 135 kg (297 lbs).

Does it not seem that this would make your child monstrously obese? That is with only 10 g (0.4 oz) extra per day. How much does a child need to eat in order to gain 10 g? It is estimated that to accumulate 1 g of body fat, a person must ingest 10.8 calories.[2] This would mean ingesting 108 kcal in order to gain 10 g. This is almost the exact amount found in one serving of strawberry yogurt, half a chocolate doughnut, one jar of baby food, or 250 ml (1 cup) of fruit juice.

Would you be happy if your child would eat one extra yogurt per day? Probably not. Many mothers prepare a whole plateful of food only to have their youngster take two bites. How much more would the child gain if he cleaned his plate every day? Twenty or thirty grams? Can you imagine your child at ten weighing 100 or 135 kg (220 to 300 lbs)?

Our metabolism allows for many important adaptations, and in reality eating one or two more bites of food may not affect our weight. But everything has a limit. Many mothers expect that their children should eat twice as much as they do as a matter of course. No one can eat twice as much as they need and remain healthy.

A child's three defences

Children have to defend themselves. If they ate everything that adults would have them eat, they would become dangerously ill. Fortunately they have a strategic defence plan against excess food, a plan they put into action automatically. Their first line of defence is to close their mouth and turn their head:

I have an eleven-month-old daughter; she has gained no weight since she was eight months. She weighed 8 kg (17 lbs 10 oz) then and weighs 8 kg now. She seems never to be hungry. We have to distract her with a toy in order to get her to eat something, but many times she turns her face and closes her mouth tight and refuses to eat at all; at that point there is no way on earth we can make her eat.

This child is communicating, much louder than if she could speak, that she does not want to eat. A wise mother would not try to force the issue. (By the way, it is not unusual for a child to stop gaining at this age, and many normal girls at this same age weigh less than 8 kg).

If mother continues to insist, the child falls back on his second line of defence: he opens his mouth but will not swallow. Liquids and strained food will leak from the corners of his mouth. Meat becomes a large fibrous lump that ends up being spat out when no more will fit in his mouth.

> *My eight-month-old son was a great eater until a week ago. One day he just started refusing to eat, at first just his afternoon fruit, and then he also refused his vegetables at lunch. His ploy is to hold food in his mouth without swallowing. At first he would hold the food for a few seconds, but he can now hold it for up to thirty minutes and I can't get him to swallow it . . .*

If she were to insist a bit more, the child might swallow some of the food. He is then left with his last weapon: throwing up.

> *My four-and-half-month-old has never had a good feeding in his entire life. I breastfed him during the first three months during which he had colic and gained very little weight; only 100 to 150 g (3.5 to 5 oz) per week. When I started bottle-feeding, he would take the first 40 to 50 ml (1.5 to 2 oz), then cried while eating and spitting up the rest, up to 100 ml (3.5 oz). I have tried giving him less, and to feed him only every three and up to four hours. I've tried to feed him when he's asleep and by distracting him with toys – nothing has worked.*
>
> *We started cereal at four months. We have had no luck. He does not eat willingly, but ingests the food because I've decided to make him eat no matter what. As a result he has started gaining much better, 250 g (9 oz) per week, but each meal is an ordeal. First I give him his bottle and, once he drinks the first 50 ml (2 oz), I start with the cereal. I have tried five different kinds of formulas and it's always the same. The only bottle nipple he accepts is the orthodontic one. Lately he has learned to make himself vomit. He doesn't even have to try hard; he just does it. It takes about an hour to feed him, on average, and I feed him five times a day.*

This child was gaining 100 to 150 g (3.5 to 5 oz) per week during the first three months and this was normal. Now at four months, he is gaining 250 g (9 oz) per week. This is not normal; it is totally excessive for his age. While it may be normal for an isolated week, it is not healthy to gain more than 1 kg (2.2 lbs) per month at this age. His only recourse is to cry and throw up. If the parents continue insisting, or if they threaten with new punishments or humiliations so he doesn't throw up, or if they resort to medication so that he can't throw up (antiemetics), then our hero is sunk.

The problem of allergies

Another reason for a child refusing to eat is that certain foods make him feel bad. Allergies to certain foods can be dangerous. Isabel's experience shows us that failure to recognize the first symptoms of allergies can lead to early weaning from the breast and can also aggravate the problem:

> *I am the mother of a seven-month-old baby who has been breastfed until now. At first everything was great and if it were up to me, I would have continued nursing much longer. It seemed to me my daughter wanted the milk to flow faster than it did, since she would nurse for five minutes and then fuss. Nursing has been very difficult these past three months, but I was sure it was best for her and I insisted she breastfeed until I could no longer stand it. Finally, I decided to wean her. I felt that breastfeeding should be a joyful event for both mother and baby and all I could see was my daughter's pain during each nursing.*
>
> *When I introduced the first bottle of formula, I was frightened to see red splotches on her face within the first few minutes. I had to breastfeed her for a few more weeks while the doctor did some allergy testing.*

The testing, as expected, came back positive. The symptoms that Isabel's daughter was showing during breastfeeding were a clear indication of allergies that no one recognized. Not even in hindsight, when the diagnosis had been confirmed, did anyone explain to Isabel the reason for her daughter's feeding behaviour.

Many mothers say that their baby "refuses the breast". A baby who was nursing well up to a few days or weeks ago suddenly only nurses five minutes or less, and then starts to cry. Two very different situations are possible:

A) The child starts to nurse happily, eats contentedly for five minutes or less, and then lets go, seemingly satiated. Since the mother has been told that the baby must nurse at least ten minutes, she thinks baby is not finished and so tries to get baby to nurse more. The baby naturally will become upset at being forced to eat.

B) The baby starts to nurse more or less happily, but seems more and more uncomfortable until he lets go of the breast in tears. Some mothers explain: "It's like the milk hits his stomach and hurts him, so he cries in pain." An excellent description since that is exactly what is going on.

The first situation is totally normal and corresponds to the normal shortening of feedings that happens as babies grow, as we will explain later (see "Crisis at three months of age" on page 98). There is nothing to do, other than to recognize that the child is finished with the feeding and to stop trying to make him nurse. If a baby is forced to take the breast for several weeks, it is possible that he may develop an aversion to the breast and may start to cry even before being forced, which would make it harder to distinguish between situation A and B. But if you think back, you might be able to remember how things started and realize that it was a classic "A" situation.

In the second situation, it is clear that the cause is allergies or intolerance to some food or medication the mother has ingested. Almost always the culprit is cow's milk, although it may also be fish, eggs, soy, citrus, or other foods. This is what happened in Isabel's case. If, at that moment, Isabel had eliminated all cow's milk from her diet, she would have saved herself a lot of tears and suffering, the alarming reaction her daughter had with the first formula bottle, the unnecessary weaning, and all the difficulties that entail feeding an allergic baby with a hypoallergenic formula (which, aside from high cost, tastes awful, causing many babies to refuse it).

Why would Isabel's daughter cry after three minutes at the breast? Some cow's milk proteins (as well as proteins from any other food that mother eats) can show up in her milk. Of course, the amount is small and it is rare to have a general reaction, with red splotches all over the body as occurred with the first formula bottle. Instead, the reaction usually occurs only in the place of contact: the oesophagus and stomach of the child. In a few minutes there is inflammation and discomfort in these places. The mother will not see a thing, but the child notices it and it hurts!

If your child shows similar symptoms to Isabel's daughter, and halfway through the feeding starts to cry as if in pain (and especially if you are seeing eczema and skin irritations as well), it would be wise to test for cow's milk allergy. To do this, the mother must keep breastfeeding while removing all milk, cheese, yogurt, butter, and all other dairy products from her diet. Become an expert label reader so you eliminate anything that has any form of milk. Bread, many desserts, chocolate and even some brands of processed lunch meat as well as many "100 percent vegetable oil" margarines contain milk products. Look for "mik", "dried milk", "milk solids", "whey", "milk serum", "milk protein", etc.

You'll have to spend seven to ten days without eating or drinking any milk products. The results are not always immediate; cow's milk proteins have been found in a mother's milk up to five days after eliminating it totally from the mother's diet. Do not substitute soymilk for cow's milk since soy triggers almost as many allergies as cow's milk.

If after ten days your child's symptoms do not improve, he was probably not allergic to cow's milk. He could be allergic to something else; you can try fish and eggs. If the symptoms are alarming and you do not wish to spend too long while you figure it out, it may be best to eliminate dairy, eggs, fish, soy and any other food that you suspect, adding them to your diet later one at a time. Some children are allergic to two or more items and they only improve when mother eliminates both at the same time. I once knew a baby who was allergic both to milk and to peaches.

Luckily the mother noticed because, when she eliminated milk, she started drinking peach juice and the child was not improving.

If the symptoms disappear after eliminating dairy products, it could be just a coincidence. Reintroduce milk to see what happens. But do not do it slowly since symptoms could be minimal and you'll have doubts. Drink two glasses of milk in one day and if nothing happens, then your child was not allergic to milk. He "got better" by coincidence, and it is best to leave it at that. It is important to do this test – the reintroduction of dairy products. Sometimes mothers are advised to eliminate all dairy products at the drop of a hat as if cow's milk was the culprit behind every baby's cries, all rashes and stuffy noses, and the mother then spends months or years without drinking milk or drinking just a bit wondering if she's hurting her child or not.

If you reintroduce milk and your child starts having the same symptoms, then you've got proof. Get ready to breastfeed as long as possible, preferably two or more years and do not give your child any cow's milk. Not with a bottle or with cereal because what happened to Isabel's daughter can happen to your child. If the child is so allergic that even a small amount in mother's milk causes problems, giving him milk directly could trigger a much more severe reaction.

Not all allergic children are so sensitive that they react when mother eats bread, pastry, or lunch meat made with a small amount of milk. In order to determine an allergy it is important to be very strict in the initial phase, just to be sure. Later on, perhaps you could eat some of these products without your child reacting negatively. It is possible that the more controlled the mother's diet is, the faster the child may outgrow the allergy, although we are not sure at this point.

If you find out that dairy products are affecting your child, talk to your doctor; he may want to do other allergy testing. And do not try to give any dairy products to your child until further notice. Warn family members and the child care facility. Children seem to outgrow milk allergies, usually at one to four years of age, but in some cases the introduction of dairy products may need to be done under a doctor's guidance, even in a hospital.

Is he really not eating a thing?

That's something else. There are eighteen-month-olds, as we have mentioned earlier, who eat less than some nine-month-olds. But there are also many that eat more, only their mother has not noticed. Nutritional knowledge does not come by divine inspiration, and it is easy to make mistakes when estimating your child's caloric intake.

One of the most frequent errors is the belief that "milk doesn't count", both mother's milk as well as other kinds. Since milk is liquid, many people see it as little more than water when, in reality, its caloric as well as protein content is very high. We have already mentioned that many baby foods, particularly vegetables, even vegetables with meat, and also most fruits, are much lower in calories than milk. Let's review Alberto's example:

My thirteen-month-old son refuses to eat fruit by itself. I can only get him to eat pureed pear or banana in a bottle and then only a small amount. He does not like juice of any kind; he rejects baby cereal, yogurt, and custards.

For breakfast, somewhere between 5 and 7 am, he drinks 240 ml (8 oz) of milk with fruit. Sometimes before lunch he will drink 180 ml (6 oz) of milk with cereal. Between noon and 1 pm he eats strained vegetables with chicken, meat, egg, or fish. Dinner consists of 210 ml (7 oz) of milk with fruit and turkey ham; he does not like cheese or anything else, only bread. Before bed, around 8:30 pm, he'll eat strained vegetables and 210 ml (7 oz) of milk with cereal.

Sweet little Alberto is drinking 840 ml (28.5 oz) of milk every day, plus fruit, strained vegetables with meat or fish, turkey cold-cuts, bread and cereal with two of his milk feedings, and his mother is worried about his intake! A thirteen-month-old baby can need up to 900 kcal per day. Just the milk alone is 590 kcal, and what about all the other food? Fortunately, the problem is about to be solved because the mother has noticed the main issue as she adds: "I no longer make him eat, since it makes things worse."

It is best for children over one year to drink no more than 500 ml (17 oz) of milk per day. If they drink more, nothing terrible will happen, but be aware that they will have little room for other foods. This is the reason that many experts recommend that bottle-fed babies be weaned from the bottle on their first birthday. Let them use a cup. It is a small trick that usually causes them to drink less milk. It is too easy to drink too much milk using a bottle.

Health professionals are not immune to this interesting belief that "milk is like water", especially when it comes to mother's milk. See what happened to Silvia:

I am the mother of a two-year-old son who is still breastfeeding. This is something that brings us both great satisfaction. He breastfeeds in spite of the opinion of doctors, family members and society. The first two months he gained weight beautifully, but since that time, we've had problems. He wouldn't nurse more than a few minutes and I have been known to nurse him while dancing around the house! He is only 10 kg (22 lbs) at two years old; however, he is healthy, strong, and very lively. The problem is that he is never hungry (doesn't know the word), and people tell me to wean him so he'll eat more since my milk is no longer nourishing – it's like "water".

I express my milk at work and freeze it. My sitter uses it to make a cereal and Meritene [concentrated protein supplement used for the ill and undernourished] shake for my son.

This is a common scenario: a baby who gains well for two months then slows down his growth while nursing much less (see "Crisis at three months of age" on page 98). And mother is made to feel that there is something wrong until she is a worried mess.

A 10 kg (22 lbs) male breastfed baby needs approximately 812 kcal per day and 8 g of protein. These are estimates made using the latest research;[4,10] many books give outdated data, with much higher numbers. In the earlier edition of this book we said 850 kcal were needed instead of 812, but newer and more precise studies by Butte have decreased the numbers again. Five ounces of human milk with one envelope of Meritene and 15 g (0.5 oz) of cereal will contain 300 calories (more than one-third of what this child needs all day) and 9 g (0.3 oz) of protein (more than he needs in a day). If he also takes in another 400 ml (14 oz) by breastfeeding, which adds 280 kcal more, plus almost 4 g (0.1 oz) of protein (plus whatever else he eats during the rest of the day), are you surprised this child is never hungry?

Many mothers think that their child does not eat because he does not eat the "required" baby foods. What they fail to notice is that their children are eating things that are the same or better. Look again at Alberto's mother's account on page 49. He eats milk with cereal two times a day and he also eats bread. However, his mother says that he refuses cereal.

This story is a great example of the mistaken belief: "If he's not eating baby food, he's not eating." A mother once came to me, in total despair: "Doctor, I can't get him to eat fruit. I have tried everything, pureed fruit, fruit with baby cereal, baby food jars, fruit yogurt, fruit Jell-O . . . nothing."

Since the child (wisely) had refused them, I didn't take the time to explain to the mother that baby cereal with fruit and fruit yogurt have very little fruit or that "fruit flavoured" yogurt and fruit Jell-O contain no fruit (only sugar and food colouring). Instead I suggested: "Sometimes babies don't like things all mushy and mixed together. Have you tried fresh fruit, like a banana or . . . ?" "Yes, I have," she interrupted. "He loves that. He will take a banana in his hand and will eat most of it. Still . . ." she insisted, "there is no way that he will take fruit."

For this mother, eating a whole banana was a waste of time since it wasn't "baby food".

Lastly, another factor that makes many mothers unaware of how much their children are eating is that they are unfamiliar with the high caloric content of some foods. Sometimes, in a desperate attempt to get the child to eat, the mother resorts to some "treat", preferably covered in chocolate. (I'm not sure what it is about chocolate, but no matter how full you feel, you can always find room for chocolate, whether you're an adult or a child). The child offered the "treat", to get him to eat, was not hungry in the first place, but he gladly accepts something sweet, and then becomes even less hungry. The fight is set to begin.

We established that a two-year-old male who weighs 10 kg (22 lbs) needs about 812 kcal per day (this is the mean, some will need much more, others much less). So if he drinks daily 500 ml (18 oz) of milk (350 kcal), eats five Oreo cookies (260 kcal), a strawberry yogurt (110 kcal), and a 200 ml (7 oz) glass of pineapple juice (85 kcal), he's eaten 805 kcal already. He will not have room for much more. What if we add a chocolate doughnut (230 kcal)? He won't be able to eat one more bite! Where do you expect him to put fruit, vegetables, meat, beans, etc? Clearly this is not an adequate diet for a two-year-old, but it has ample calories and the child won't be able to eat anything else.

Therefore, if you want your child to eat healthy foods, you must stop giving him "treats". Limit milk and dairy products to no more than 500 ml (17 oz) or less a day for children older than twelve months, don't offer anything but water to drink (no more milk, juice, and never any fizzy drinks), and save the treats for special occasions such as holidays or birthdays.

Chapter 2
Your child knows what she or he needs

All animals in the world know what they need. While walking in the countryside you don't find a creature on the side of the road dead because no one told it what to eat. Each creature chooses an appropriate diet for its species; it's as hard to find a rabbit eating meat, as it is to find a wolf eating grass.

Most human adults also eat what they need without being told. People who exercise regularly eat more, and those who lead more sedentary lives eat less without having an expert come in to calculate caloric intake and give them written instructions. Sure, some of us have a propensity toward obesity, but when we stop to think about what could happen and doesn't, we realize that the system that controls our food intake is actually quite good. If every day you were to eat a little more than you should, enough to gain 20 g (0.7 oz) per day, after a year you would have gained 7.3 kg (16 lbs) and 73 kg (160 lbs) in ten years (above what you weigh right now!). If, on the other hand, you were to lose 20 g per day, in eight or nine years you would have completely disappeared, leaving behind just a pile of empty clothing, like in the movies. Yet many people manage to weigh about the same, give or take a few pounds, over dozens of years.

The same is true in terms of the quality of your diet. Most common mortals do not know what vitamins they need, nor do they care to know what amounts they need of each or which foods contain the required nutrients (sure, you know that oranges have vitamin C, but where can you find vitamins B_1, B_{12}, or folic acid?). In spite of this, it is very rare, unless someone is truly starving, for anyone to suffer from scurvy, beriberi, anaemia, or xerophthalmia.

So how do we manage? Each person, each creature, has innate mechanisms that cause him to look for the foods he needs and to eat the right amounts. What makes us think that our children lack these same mechanisms? The young of other species have them. If a child is allowed to eat what he wants, it makes sense that he will eat what he needs. But if logical arguments are not enough to convince you of this, perhaps you'd be interested to know that this is not only logical, but scientifically proven. In the next section we will explain how children choose their food from birth, changing the composition of human milk, and how, after a few months, they are able to choose for themselves an adequate diet.

Breastfeeding "a la carte": why not to keep a regular schedule

Breastfeeding schedules are a myth. There was a time when it was thought that babies had to nurse every three hours, or every four hours, and for exactly ten minutes on each side! Have you ever wondered why for ten minutes, and not nine or eleven? Apparently these are round numbers. So how did we come to believe that a "round number" was an "exact number"?

Of course, adults never eat "ten minutes from each plate every four hours". How long do we take to finish our plate? Well, that would depend on how fast we eat! Children are the same. If they nurse fast, they may spend less than ten minutes, and if they nurse slowly, they will take longer.[11]

We do eat at set hours, but only because job obligations force us to organize our schedules in this way. Usually, when we have a day off, we skip our usual routine without damaging our health in the least. However, there are still people out there who believe babies have to get used to a schedule and they make vague references to discipline or good digestion.

For an adult, food can wait. Our metabolism allows us to wait for a meal, and the food will be the same now or in an hour's time. But your child cannot wait. His hunger pangs are urgent and his food changes if the meal gets delayed. Human milk is not a dead food, but a living tissue in the process of constant change. The amount of fat in the milk increases as the feeding progresses. The first milk is low in fat, and the milk toward the end of a feeding is higher in fat; it may be up to five times higher.

The average amount of fat at any particular feeding will depend on four factors: it will decrease the longer it has been since the last feeding (longer interval, lower fat); and it will increase with the concentration of fat toward the end of the previous feeding, the amount of milk the baby ingested at the previous feeding, and the amount he is ingesting at the present feeding. According to the excellent review by Woolridge on the physiology of breastfeeding,[12] these are the four factors that influence the fat content of the milk:

1. Interval from the previous feeding,
2. Fat concentrations at the end of the previous feeding,
3. Amount of milk taken at the previous feeding,
4. Amount of milk taken at this feeding.

When the child takes both sides, he rarely empties the second breast. We could simplify this and say that he drinks two-thirds skim milk and one-third cream. However, the child who only takes one breast per feeding can be said to take in half skim milk, half cream. If he takes lower fat milk (and therefore, fewer calories), the baby may accept greater volume, and therefore consume more protein. In effect, the baby who drinks 50 ml (1.5 oz) from each side is not taking in the same as the one who takes in 100 ml (3 oz) from just one breast; and the diet of the baby who takes in 80 ml (2.7 oz) every two hours will be totally different from the diet of the baby who drinks 160 ml (5.4 oz) every four hours.

The controlling factors in milk composition are still being studied and what we don't know is still probably greater than what we do know. For example, it has been noted that one breast often produces more milk, with a higher protein concentration than the other one. Maybe this is just coincidence, or perhaps your child can choose, by nursing more on one side or the other, a meal with more or less protein.

And you thought your baby always ate the same thing? Did you imagine it was boring to spend months drinking only milk? Well, this is not so with mother's milk. Your child has at his disposal a large selection of "menu" items from which to choose, from a light soup to creamy dessert. Since the baby can't talk (nor could the breast understand him, for that matter), the baby puts in his order in three ways:

1. By the **amount of milk** he drinks at each feeding (that is, nursing for a shorter or longer amount of time, and with more or less intensity).
2. The **interval** between one feeding and the next.
3. Drinking from **one or both breasts**.

What your child does at the breast to obtain exactly what he needs from one day to the next is pure engineering. The child has total and perfect control over his diet as long as he can change the variables at will. This is what feeding on demand means: let the baby decide when he wants to nurse, how long he wants to be at the breast, and if he wants one or both sides.

When a child is not allowed to control one of the mechanisms, most of the time he manages an adequate diet by manoeuvring the other two variables. In one experiment,[13] some babies were kept on only one breast per feeding for one week, and on two breasts the following week (the order of which week was random). In theory, the babies would have ingested much more fat during the days when they were kept on only one side than when they were offered both sides. However, the babies spontaneously modified the frequency and duration of their feedings and were able to take in similar amounts of fat (but different volumes of milk).

But if a baby is not allowed to modify the frequency or the duration of the feedings, and is not allowed to decide if he wants to nurse on one side or both, he is lost. He will not drink the milk he needs, but is stuck with whatever he gets. If his diet is too far removed from his real needs, he will have problems gaining weight appropriately, or he will spend the day hungry and fussy. This is why breastfeeding on a schedule rarely works and the stricter the schedule, the more catastrophic the result. Babies need to nurse irregularly; only then can they get a balanced diet.

From his very first day, though he seemed to be only drinking milk, your child has been choosing his diet from a wide array of choices, and he has always chosen wisely, both in quantity and in quality.

Solids also "a la carte"

In the 1920s, Dr. Adelle Davis demonstrated through a series of experiments, that children could choose a balanced diet for themselves.[14] She took a group of children, ranging in ages from six to eighteen months, and offered them ten or twelve different foods at each meal. The foods were unmixed: carrots, rice, chicken, eggs . . . Children would eat as much as they wanted of whatever they wanted without any adult control. The older ones fed themselves while the younger ones were spoon-fed by an adult who would offer each of the different foods without insistence, starting with one food at a time until the child closed his mouth, then moving on to the next food until all the foods were offered. Over the next several months, these children's growth was normal and their intake of nutrients adequate on average, although the variations from meal to meal were "a nutritionist's nightmare". Children would sometimes eat "like a bird" and sometimes "like a horse"; they would have food jags where they only ate one or two items for days at a time, only to forget about those foods a few days later. Yet one way or another, they all finally managed to eat a balanced diet.

Other, more modern studies have confirmed that small children, when allowed to eat what they wish, both in the laboratory[15] as well as at home,[16] will take in a consistent amount of calories from day to day, although variations between meals are wide.

But won't he stuff himself with chocolate?

Sure! If he is allowed. Or at least that is what we think would happen although there are no scientific studies that demonstrate this. It could also be that he would stuff himself the first day and when he got tired of chocolate he would still eat a balanced diet. Children (and adults) show preference for sweet and salty foods, and we tend to overeat both of these foods. If children possess an innate mechanism that tells them to eat what they need, why do children love to eat "junk food"?

To understand why the control mechanism sometimes fails, we need to keep in mind the theory of evolution. When an animal is healthy, it lives longer and has more offspring; therefore, natural selection favours those animals that show healthy feeding behaviours. But natural selection takes many years to work and the behaviour that was valuable at one point may no longer be so good if living conditions change.

What good was a preference for sweet and salty foods for the cave children of Altamira in Spain? Not only did they lack chocolate, they also lacked salt or sugar. The sweetest thing they had was mother's milk, their main food source, and fruit, which is full of vitamins. The saltiest food was probably meat, an important source of iron and protein. Their preferences, therefore, helped them choose a varied and balanced diet. But now we have sweets that are much sweeter than fruit, and snacks much saltier than meat, and our selection mechanism has gone a little haywire.

Even so, it is surprising how strong the instinct to choose a healthy diet really is. Just look at advertising: the less healthy a food is, the more they need to advertise it. Some brands of salty snacks, sweets and soda, though they already sell millions, keep advertising daily. They know that they cannot rest for one moment, for if they did not advertise, their sales would show a huge drop. On the other hand, lentils, apples, rice, or bread do not need to be advertised much at all and people still eat them.

Just in case, though, experts[14] suggest that children can choose a healthy diet, on the condition that we offer them healthy alternatives. If you offer your child fruit, pasta, chicken and peas, and then let him choose what and how much to eat, he will certainly, over time, choose an adequate diet – even if he may eat only peas one day, then only chicken on the next two days. But if you give him a choice between fruit, pasta, peas, and chocolate, then no one is guaranteeing that he will have a balanced diet.

In brief, it is the parents' only responsibility to offer a variety of healthy foods. It is up to the child to choose among these foods what he eats and how much.

Chapter 3
What *not* to do at mealtimes

When it comes to getting children to eat, mothers' creativity knows no limits (although fathers often participate less in this, it is probably more because of indifference than conscious planning). It all begins by make-believing that the spoon is an airplane. Then come distractions (or "tricking", a word which many mothers use without remorse): songs, dancing, toys, or the inevitable television. Begging soon follows ("Don't do this to mummy!"), promises ("When you finish eating, then you can play"), then threats ("If you don't finish your dinner, you won't get to play"), supplications ("One for mummy, one for daddy, one for granny"), and comparisons ("Don't you want to be strong like Popeye?"). It is said that when one couple observed their child eating everything she could find on the floor, they had a brilliant idea. After washing the floor spick and span, they would spread bits of potato omelette for the child to eat.

Some of the methods make us laugh, but some move us to tears, especially the child. Let's see some examples.

Patience?

My son is five months old and he won't take a spoon. I started trying at four months but no matter how hard I tried (with much patience), the child would cry, spit food out and fuss. So I had to put the baby food in the bottle. Now he will accept four to six bites without fussing, but then, that's it! I have started putting the pacifier in his mouth after each bite of food and that's the only way he will finish everything.

Patience? This is another misconception. Patience would have been to accept that this baby was not ready for solids. This mother has not been patient at all, but merciless. (If the baby could talk, he would probably use a much stronger word; "pushy" would be the nicest.) To put a pacifier in after every bite is a dirty trick. The child's sucking reflex makes him swallow instead of spitting it out. It seems to have worked for a couple of days, but it won't last for long. The child would get sick if he kept eating like this for long, and nature rarely lets this happen. He will find a way to spit the food out, with or without the pacifier, or he will learn to throw up.

Night raids

My daughter is thirteen months old and she has this strange behaviour at mealtimes. She will not eat. I offer different things, and she will not even try them; it's like she's afraid of food. But the strangest thing is that if I offer her a bottle, she also refuses, but if I go in while she's asleep, she drinks it all down (with cereal), she drinks 600 to 700 ml (20 to 24 oz) of milk in 24 hours. She never seems to be hungry. Can a child who has never been forced to eat hate food?

Never been forced to eat? What do you call forcing down more than 500 ml of milk with cereal during sleep? Of course, people don't tie their children down. When we talk about making or forcing a child to eat, we are talking about all the methods, both the harsh ones and the "gentle" ones. By the way, how can you expect this child to be hungry during the day when she's had more than half a litre of milk and cereal during the night? She has room for nothing else.

Those hateful comparisons

According to a well-known apocryphal story, Cain was a "bad eater". While doing "the airplane" (or was it the pterodactyl?) with the spoon, Eve would encourage him saying: "Be a good boy, Cain, look at your brother, Abel. He's finished all his veggies." You do know the end of that story, right?

We are seldom aware how badly comparisons make our children feel. The child who is being used as the example is also bothered. "Look how Monica has finished her plate." Our daughter is furious and poor Monica is thinking, "Get me out of here, please!"

Would you like this to be done to you? Imagine you are having coffee with your best friend. In comes your husband who says, "I'd like to see you take care of your appearance for once. See how Encarna has done her hair and face, and how thin she looks. You always look like a slob." Then he leaves, happy as a clam, and you are left there with Encarna. Which of you would be the first to open your mouth now?

As a father, I've been embarrassed when giving my children their lunch at school. Occasionally some mother decides to make my daughters an example: "Look at the big sandwich that she's eating for lunch." What am I supposed to do? Do I pretend not to hear and get out of there as soon as possible? Or do I stay and explain that she'll eat the sandwich if she wants it, that sometimes she only eats half, and that sometimes she doesn't even touch it. Or shall I explain that whatever she doesn't eat will become my snack?

Bribes

Many desperate parents resort to "bribing" their child to get them to eat. Dr. Illingworth, whose book we have already quoted, mentions the case of a child who amassed an extensive collection of matchbox cars in this way.[1]

Curiously enough, someone has bothered to research the

effectiveness of bribes. In one study[14] a new food was offered to two groups of children. One group was promised a prize if they tried the new food. The other group was simply faced with the new food to do whatever they wanted. A few days later, the children in the prize group were eating less of the new food than the other group. You would have to be a fool not to figure out that "It must not be very good if they offer me a prize in order to try it."

Neither is it a good idea to use food as a prize or punishment. "If you are a good boy, I'll buy you an ice cream" or "You hit your cousin so there will be no dessert for you." I believe this is a dietary mistake on top of a child-rearing one. In the first place, even if the prize were a toy and the punishment meant not going to the circus, I don't think that this is the best way to teach a child. A child will do what is right because of the satisfaction that this brings, and he does not need more reward than the approval of his parents (and soon, not even that, because he'll have his own approval, which is most important); he will abstain from behaving badly when he understands that this hurts other people. Good people, those with a higher moral conscience (and little children have this, no doubt about it), do not need rewards or punishments. An adult who only acts because he hopes for a reward or fears punishment will be a hypocrite and an opportunist, doing what is right when being observed and doing what is wrong in secret. When you take your child to the zoo, don't spoil the occasion with phrases such as, "We're here because this week you picked up all your toys." This phrase is a lie and you know it. You know perfectly well that you'd be going to the zoo anyway, that you take him because you care about him. Because he is your child, you love him unconditionally; you want to make him happy and to enjoy your weekend together. Why should you hide your love from your child and pretend that the outing is just a reward?

Going back to food, in addition to the child-rearing dilemma with which you may or may not agree, to use food as a reward or punishment adds a nutritional problem. Because the prize will never be Swiss chard, and the punishment will never be chocolate. The opposite will be true, idealizing once again the kinds of foods that your child must not overeat.

The most ridiculous situation, if you really stop to think about it, is the one that goes: "If you don't finish your peas, you can't have cake." Every time I hear that, I have the hardest time not laughing. If the child is not hungry anymore, how do you expect that on top of the peas, he'll eat cake? The logical statement should be: "Since you've eaten lots of peas, it's better if you skip dessert", or maybe, "You better stop eating peas, don't forget we have cake."

Research has proven that when children are around a certain food, but are not allowed to eat it, they want it all the more.[17] In other words, if you have sweets at home, and spend all day saying "no more sweets", you'll only manage to have your children ask for sweets all the more. If you want your child to stay away from sweets, it's probably best not to have them at home, and then you won't have to mention them at all.

Appetite stimulants

Our baby is almost eleven months old and we are so worried about him. Since he was born, he has never been a good eater (he only breastfed for six weeks) and by three months old we had to give him his formula with a spoon because he wouldn't drink from the bottle and that's the only way we could get him to eat. When he was five months old, I took him to a new doctor who prescribed an appetite stimulant. This worked wonders for six weeks, but once we stopped the medication, we went back to the same problem. Then, at nine months, we tried the medicine again and, although it didn't work as well as the first time, he did improve a bit. But now that we've stopped giving it to him, he is worse than ever. He's doing what he'd never done before; he is throwing up. He also gags on the spoon (even the first bite). He has been throwing up every day. If it's not at breakfast, then it's at lunch; if not then, it's at the mid-afternoon feeding. If we are lucky and he made it through most of the day without incident, then certainly he will throw up at dinner. Mealtimes have become pure hell. His mother, who spends most of the time with him, now needs a therapist for herself; she is so worried about all these food issues, believing he won't grow like the other children unless this problem is solved.

There are two types of appetite stimulants on the market: the ones that work and those that do not.

1. The ones that **do not work** are unbelievable combinations of vitamins and strange ingredients, usually with an impressive name that makes mention of metabolism, growth, energy, or something along those lines. They are the modern equivalent of that famous "Dr. McWhomever's Good-for-Everything Snake Oil Tonic" that quacks are seen selling in old Western movies. (Some of these modern remedies still have alcohol in them just as they did years ago.)

In small doses and for short-term use they are generally harmless; but they are not always totally safe. There may be an allergic reaction to any of the components, additives, or colourings, and some plants with "stimulant" effects (such as ginseng) have been known to be toxic. Also, some vitamins and minerals can also be toxic if consumed in large enough quantities.

Most doctors agree that these "tonics" are absolutely useless, but some will recommend them as a placebo. A placebo (from the Latin "I shall please") is a false medication given to the patient to keep him happy. Sometimes, giving the child a prescription to "keep the parents happy" is easier and quicker than explaining the truth. It is also true that some patients demand medication and sometimes the doctor has to give in and recommend a harmless placebo for fear that the patient may go out on his own and buy his own medication at great risk. (Unfortunately, in Spain it is very easy to obtain medications without a prescription.) By the way, if you don't want to be given placebos, in this or other situations, it's good to tell the doctor up front and to remind him from time to time: "I don't like giving my child medications unless they are needed; if you think that he will get better on his own, you don't have to prescribe anything." Many doctors will respond with a wide appreciative smile.

2. The ones that **do work** are in another category. They almost always contain cyproheptadine (combined with diverse vitamins to distinguish one brand from the next).

It is important to note that hunger is not in the stomach, just as love is not in the heart. Appetite is in (or is controlled by) the brain. Cyproheptadine (or some cousin to it like dihexazin) acts on the brain appetite centre, just like sleeping pills work on the brain sleep centre. Cyproheptadine is a **psychoactive** drug and its side effects are: drowsiness (a frequent side effect that can impact school performance), dry mouth, headaches, nausea and, rarely, high blood pressure, agitation, confusion or hallucinations, and decreased secretion of human growth hormone (so the child will be short and fat, to round out the successful treatment!). Intoxication (should the child find the bottle and decide to swallow all of it) can produce a deep sleep, weakness or loss of muscle coordination, convulsions and fever.

Of course, these serious side effects are rare; I don't mention them to scare you if you've ever given these medications to your child. (If we told you all the possible side effects for common medications like amoxicillin or acetaminophen, you'd also get scared.) Any time you take medication you are taking a risk; what you need to keep in mind is that, when you are sick and in need of the medication, that risk is much smaller than the benefit you would derive from taking the drug. The problem with appetite stimulants is that the children who take them are neither sick nor do they need the treatment; the benefit is nil, and any risk, as small or remote as it may be, is unacceptable.

Without a doubt, the greatest danger of cyproheptadine is that it does work; the child eats more. More than he needs, more than is healthy. Fortunately, the effect goes away when the medication is stopped and most children will start to lose any weight they had gained while on the medication. This "rebound effect" often shows the parents the futility of using the medicine and most will stop using it. But some parents are tempted and will use it continuously, for months and years. What effect can overeating for months or years, combined with decreased physical activity due to drowsiness, bring? Certainly nothing good.

Herbs and other "natural" products have also been used to make children eat. All of these products, no matter how "natural" they are, can also be classified in one of the two previous groups: those that work and those that don't (the problem is that we sometimes lack the necessary information to distinguish between the two). If they do not work, why waste your time and money? And if they do work, their dangers will be similar to those of cyproheptadine. First, because if they do increase appetite, they probably affect the brain. Second, because you can't make a child eat more than he needs without damaging his health long-term.

Fortunately, it seems that the alcoholic preparations that were used years ago to increase appetite have gone out of fashion. It should go without saying: never give alcohol to a child.

I can't emphasize this enough: appetite stimulants are worthless when they don't work and dangerous when they do, their effect is temporary and they have rebound effects. They should never be used.

Firsthand account

If our children could talk, what would they say? Perhaps something along these lines:

> *Since I turned nine months old I started to notice my parents becoming so pushy about food. Up until now, they fed me quite well; but then they started wanting to give me one more bite when I was already finished, and one day they tried to get me to eat something repugnant and gelatinous, which they called liver. They said it was very good for me. At first these were isolated incidents and I didn't pay much attention to them. Sometimes, just to make them happy, I would eat an extra bite even though I would find myself feeling stuffed all afternoon and had to eat a little less at the next feeding. I now regret what I've done and think I should have stood my ground from the start. I wonder if it's true what people say – that if you give in to your parents even one time, you spoil them and then they become too demanding?*

I always thought I would raise my parents with patience and dialogue, far removed from the authoritarianism of the past. But now, in light of what has happened, I don't know what to think.

The real problems started about six weeks ago, when I was ten months old. Quite suddenly I started to feel ill. My head, back and throat hurt. My head was the worst. Any noise would resound and reverberate all through my body from the top of my head to the tips of my toes. When grandma would call me "Cuchi Cuchi" (she always calls me that, and I almost like it better than Jonathan), it felt like my head was about to explode. To make things worse, instead of being able to let it all out by crying like I usually do, my own cries would resonate in my head and make me feel worse. That mushy stuff that comes out in my diaper sometimes (I don't know what it is, but mummy never lets me play with it) also changed; it smelled bad and burned my bottom. My friend from the playground, Alberto, who is thirteen months old, told me that I had a virus and that I would get better soon, but my parents must not know so much as Alberto, because they looked so worried. They acted as if they didn't know what to do.

For a whole week I couldn't even swallow. Good thing I still had the breast; that always goes down easy, but solids were another story. I felt such a lump in my throat that I ended up throwing up. The weird thing was, I wasn't even hungry. I would tell my parents what was happening, but they just didn't get it. Sometimes I get so frustrated with them. I think it's time for them to learn my language. They get everything backwards. I would cry quietly and for a long time saying, "Hold me" and they would just put me in the crib. I would pout to say, "Today I don't want to eat" and they just brought me more food.

I would twist my face protesting, "One more bite and I'll vomit" and they got all mad and started shouting at me something about "misbehaving".

Good thing the headache only lasted a few days. But my parents have not been the same since. They keep insisting I eat food I don't want. And no longer just one more bite as before: now they expect me to eat twice or three times as much as before.

They are acting very strangely; one minute they are euphoric, making fools of themselves with a spoon, yelling, "Look at the airplane, brrrrooom!"; then they get mad and start trying to get me to open my mouth or they get emotional and weepy. I wonder if they caught the virus. Perhaps their head and back hurt too. Whatever it is, now mealtimes are a huge ordeal. Just the thought of them makes me want to throw up and I lose what little appetite I had.

Chapter 4
Feeding guides

It is impossible to give detailed recommendations on infants' and young children's feeding that are based on science. Although committees of experts have tackled the topic, their recommendations have been extremely cautious and their conclusions are very non-specific.

Recommendations from ESPGAN

In Europe, people usually follow the guidelines set forth by the European Society of Paediatric Gastroenterology and Nutrition (ESPGAN), published in 1982.[18] After reviewing hundreds of scientific research studies, experts from nine countries gave the following seven recommendations.

1. In giving advice note should be taken of the sociocultural milieu of the family, the attitude of the parents, and the quality of the motherchild relationship.
2. In general *Beikost* [anything that the baby eats aside from mother's milk or artificial baby milk] should not be introduced earlier than 3 months nor later than 6 months. It should be started in small amounts and both the variety and quantity should be increased slowly.
3. By the age of 6 months not more than 50% of the energy

content should derive from *Beikost*. For the remainder of the first year breast milk, formula, or equivalent dairy products should be given in a quantity of not less than 500 ml [17 oz] daily.

4. There is no need to specify the type of *Beikost* (cereals, fruits, vegetables) to be introduced first. In this respect national habits and economic factors should be considered. It is not necessary to make detailed recommendation regarding the age when non-milk animal protein should be started, but the introduction of certain foods known to be highly allergenic such as eggs and fish is propably best defered until 5-6 months.

5. Gluten containing foods should not be introduced before 4 months of age. Even further postponement until the age of 6 months may be advisable.

6. Foods with a potentially high nitrate content such as spinach or beetroot should be avoided during the early months.

7. Special consideration should be given to the introduction of *Beikost* to infants with a family history of atopy in whom potentially highly allergenic foods should be strictly avoided during the first year.

Even though the ESPGAN recommendations were written in English, they use the German word *Beikost* to refer to anything that the baby eats aside from mother's milk or artificial baby milk. It therefore includes juices and teas, strained foods, teething biscuits, bottles thickened with cereal, or a bite of sausage. The expression would be equivalent to "complementary foods" which traditionally are referred to as solids in English. Unfortunately, when seeing the word "solids" there is always some poor soul who takes it literally: "See, it says no solids until six months, but it doesn't say anything about liquids. Juice and cereal in the bottle must be started much sooner." We must keep in mind that the term "solids" also refers to liquids and strained foods, just as "first foods" may or may not be strained food. There should be nothing added to babies' diets before six months, not cereal in a bottle, not juice, not tea . . . nothing.

In 2008, the ESPGHAN (an 'H' for hepatology has been added) published a new document.[19] Its recommendations are:

- Exclusive or full breast-feeding for about 6 months is a desirable goal. Complementary feeding should not be introduced in any infant before 17 weeks, and all infants should start complementary feeding by 26 weeks.
- The term "complementary feeding" should embrace all solid foods and liquids other than breast milk or infant formula and follow-on formula. The Committee suggests that including HMS [human milk substitutes] as complementary foods is unhelpful and even confusing.
- Although there are theoretical reasons why different complementary foods may have particular benefits for breast-fed or formula-fed infants, the Committee considers that attempts to devise and implement separate recommendations for breast-fed and formula-fed infants may present considerable practical difficulties and are therefore undesirable.
- Avoidance or delayed introduction of potentially allergenic foods, such as fish and eggs, has not been convincingly shown to reduce allergies, either in infants considered at risk for the development of allergy or in those not considered to be at risk.
- During the complementary feeding period, >90% of the iron requirements of a breast-fed infant must be met by complementary foods. These should provide sufficient bioavailable iron.
- Cow's milk is a poor iron source. It should not be used as the main drink before 12 months, although small volumes may be added to complementary foods.
- It is prudent to avoid both early (<4 months) and late ($\geq$ 7 months) introduction of gluten and to introduce gluten gradually while the infant is still breast-fed because this may reduce the risk of CD, type 1 diabetes mellitus, and wheat allergy.
- Infants and young children receiving a vegetarian diet should

receive a sufficient amount (~500 ml) of milk (breast milk or formula) and dairy products.
- Infants and young children should not receive a vegan diet.

Admittedly, as a final summary, it is not very specific. In the text are some other recommendations that have not made it to the final list:

- Introduce foods one at a time.
- Introduce lumpy solid foods before ten months.
- Do not add salt and sugar, avoid frequent consumption of juice (for their excess sugar).

Recommendations from the AAP

In 1981, the American Academy of Pediatrics (AAP) published some recommendations on infant feeding.[20] Much like the European ones, the AAP guidelines do not give a detailed recommendation on the order or amount of different foods. Introduction of new foods does not take place by the calendar, but more in terms of the baby's development. The baby is ready to start other foods when:

- He can sit without help. (It would be hard to feed a child that keeps falling to the side.)
- He has lost the tongue thrust reflex, which is what makes babies spit out a spoon with their tongues. This reflex probably was originally intended to keep babies from eating flies, rocks and other nasty things; at least until they were old enough to know what's food and what's not. There is nothing quite as sad as watching a mother trying to feed a baby who has not lost its tongue thrust reflex. There is food on the bib, on the diaper, in the child's hair, in the mother's hair, on the chair, on the floor – everywhere except in the little darling's mouth.
- He shows interest in adults' food. One of these days, when watching you eat, your baby will try to get some food for himself.

- He can show hunger and satiety through gestures. When he sees the spoon coming, the hungry child opens his mouth and leans forward. The child who is full will close his mouth and turn his head. This way mother knows that the child has finished eating. If the baby is too young to show satiety clearly, you run the risk of unintentionally overfeeding. Given that you should never, ever, ever make a child eat, you should not feed a baby who can't refuse to eat when full.

The AAP also insists on introducing new foods one at a time, in small quantities, and with at least a week in between new foods. This is so you can see if the baby tolerates a new food well or not.

The 1981 norms are now obsolete, and the AAP no longer includes them in their current advice, yet they haven't replaced them with others of the same level. Perhaps this is because the AAP considers the subject of little importance: children can be fed without the need for any official advice.

However, the AAP's advice on breastfeeding is up to date,[21] and as far as we are concerned ratifies that of 1997.[22] As for complementary feeding, it recommends:

- Exclusive breastfeeding, on demand, for six months.
- Gradual introduction of solid foods (specially those that are rich in iron) in the second half of the first year, complementing the human milk diet which should continue for at least 12 months, and thereafter for as long as mutually desired.

Recommendations from the WHO and UNICEF

Among other things, the World Health Organization (WHO) and the United Nations Children's Fund (UNICEF) recommend:[23]

- Exclusive breastfeeding for six months.
- Try additional foods from the age of approximately six months on.
- Continued breastfeeding, along with appropriate comp-

lementary foods up to two years and beyond.
- Offer a variety of foods.
- Until the age of twelve months, offer the breast before other foods, to ensure adequate milk intake.
- Children younger than three must eat five to six times per day (minimum).
- Offer preferably foods rich in energy (calories), iron and vitamin A. If needed, add oil or butter to vegetables to increase the caloric load (of course, should olive oil be available, this is preferable to butter or other oils).

Science fiction and infant feeding

As we can see, recommendations from experts the world over are not at all detailed. There is no clue as to the order in which different foods should be introduced, or at what age to introduce them, much less their amounts, the times of day, or days of the week when they should be offered to baby. However, it is easy to find incredibly detailed feeding guides. For example:

"At 1:00 pm, give a mixture of strained cooked potarrots (50 g), casquash (30 g), and green bays (30 g). On Monday, Wednesday, and Friday, add half a parrot breast; on Tuesday, Thursday, and Saturday, add calf sliver (50 g)…"

"At 5:00 pm, half a kweary fruit, half a panana, one-fourth bapple mixed with one-fourth cup of prungerine juice…"

We have used fictitious food names to avoid having a mother who might be skimming this book start taking notes about what to feed her baby.

You may have heard or read similar instructions. You may have even tried following them at some point. Have you ever wondered why, for example, they recommend fruit in the afternoon and not in the morning? Why 50 g (1.7 oz) of potatoes and not 40 g (1.4 oz)? Cereal at six months, fruit at seven, or fruit first and then cereal? Half of a large banana, or half of a small banana? Why half a pear and half an apple, why not a whole apple one day and a whole pear the next?

If a mother ever tried to voice a question like this, she might have received a firm "Because that's the way to do it", or even a reassuring "It really doesn't matter", or maybe a silent stare. Some mothers have heard some truly novel answers.

One friend of mine from France (now living in Spain) asked her doctor why she had to combine five fruits in the same mix for her baby, because in her country (at least in her town) they normally offered one different fruit per day. "This is a perfectly balanced mixture" was the answer she received.

At other times we have heard that cereals must be mixed with milk because if they are mixed with water, their caloric density (the amount of calories per ml) would be too low. It's a plausible explanation, but it leaves some questions unanswered: why then, should we not add milk to fruit or vegetables, whose caloric density is much lower than that of cereals?

Curiously, these detailed recommendations never match each other. They have not been able to match throughout history (see the Appendix "A bit of history" on page 166) and they don't match now. In different books, different countries, different cities and different neighbourhoods, feeding charts are totally different. I knew of a paediatric practice that had four doctors. The nurses were in charge of giving out the written instructions for infant feeding. "Who is your doctor?" they would ask before giving out the sheets. There were four different sheets!

Why don't the true experts give us more detailed instructions about child and infant feeding? Because they can only give recommendations that are evidence-based. Maybe not definitive, watertight evidence – and maybe subject to revision pending new research – but at least some kind of evidence.

We say, for example, that exclusively breastfed babies do not need to drink extra water because in several research studies done in warm climates, including deserts, it has been proven that on-demand breastfed babies do just fine without drinking water. We also say that "baby infusions" (those little pouches with powder that are mixed with water to make "tea" in many countries) are bad for babies because we've documented hundreds of cases of severe dental caries caused by these high-sugar drinks.

We recommend exclusive breastfeeding for six months because in a research study[24] babies were divided at random into two groups. One group was exclusively breastfed until six months, and then started solids (with continued breastfeeding). The other group started solids at four months. The group that started solids earlier did not grow faster, nor were any other advantages noted; but it was noted that they breastfed less. We still have not done a research study comparing solids at six versus eight months, so we may yet be in for a surprise in the future.

We say that gluten-containing food should be introduced slowly and in small amounts because it has been seen that, when introduced too quickly, some children have severe attacks of celiac disease (an intestinal illness that is worse the earlier it starts).

We say to hold off on foods that tend to be most allergenic (like milk, eggs, fish and soy) because we have seen that, when these foods are introduced early, the risk of developing allergies increases.

But, what research do we have to recommend cereal before fruit, or vice versa? None. Only the personal opinions of different people: "I believe we must start with cereal because it is higher in protein." "Nonsense, fruit must come first, it is higher in vitamin C."

To know for sure, we would have to run an experiment: give fifty children fruit first, and another fifty cereal, and then see what happens. Of course, all their other foods and circumstances must be identical.

No one has yet done this experiment. And it is unlikely that anyone will ever do it.

Let's suppose that someone does the experiment. What would be our measurable result? Infant mortality? Of course not. No child will die with either of these diets. Would it change the rate of allergies? That might work if we were to compare fruit and fish, which has been done, and that is why we wait to offer fish. But between cereal and fruit, as far as we know, there will not be much difference in terms of allergies. What food do they like best, will take more of, which do they throw up less? Supposing there are differences, they will be individual; some will prefer fruit, others cereal. It is best to do your own trial and give your child what he likes, and not what 70 percent of children in some experiment liked.

Of course, not all effects will be seen short term. If we wait a few months, maybe some differences will be evident among the groups. Maybe at a year old, one group may weigh more than the other, for example. But this leaves us with a difficult question: is the diet that makes babies heavier better because it avoids malnutrition, or is the diet that makes babies leaner better because it prevents obesity? In the majority of the world, the biggest problem is malnutrition, but in industrialized nations, almost no one dies from malnutrition, while obesity is at an epidemic rate, with severe health consequences.

Perhaps what we should measure is overall health, not weight. Shall we wait a few more months to see who walks first, or who talks sooner or with a larger vocabulary? And what good is it to start talking sooner, if, later at school, you get suspended for talking in class? And what good is it to get good grades at school if then you can't find a job? After a few years, will diet really influence health? Will these individuals have higher or lower cholesterol, more or less cancer, more or fewer heart attacks?

After all is said and done, our scientific experiment can last 30 or 50 years and we probably will not find an important difference between either starting fruit or starting cereal first. Or maybe we will find a difference, and then we'll have another problem: what to do with the results?

Let's imagine, for example (everything continues to be make-believe) that children who start fruit first weighed 150 g (5.2 oz) more at one year than those who started with cereal; that they walked three weeks earlier; their math scores at ten years old were lower, but their social studies scores at age fifteen were higher; they had fewer heart attacks at age twenty-five but had lower paying jobs; they had higher cholesterol but lower blood pressure; their stomach cancer rate was 15 percent higher at age forty, but at fifty their rate for arthritis was 20 percent lower.

Being the mother and having all this data in hand (supposing it is all trustworthy and proven), you must still choose: do you start with fruit or cereal?

We have been somewhat pessimistic. We have first supposed that no important difference was found, and then we have imagined that significant differences do exist but cancel each other out. There is a third possibility (although remote): that our study will find clear differences between both diets. Let's suppose that it had been proven scientifically, beyond a doubt, that those who start out eating fruit are more healthy, good looking, smart, and happy for their entire life than those who start with cereal. Finding this out has taken us more than fifty years. We proudly and happily announce our results to the world. And instead of being showered with gratitude, we are pummelled with a multitude of new questions: what if we start vegetables first, or chicken? Shall we start at six, seven, or seven and a half months? Shall we start with apple, pear, or banana? We don't grow apples and pears in our country; can we start with mango, pineapple, or papaya? Half an apple or a whole one? Golden, Gala, or Red Delicious? Are the vitamins the same if the fruit has been just picked or what if they've been refrigerated? Should I include the skin, since it does have more vitamins, or peel it since it contains pesticides? We would have to start a whole new study to respond to each of these questions.

This is why we started out by saying that these studies have never been done and will never be done. We will never have the answer.

Part II
What to do if your child won't eat

Chapter 5
An experiment that will change your life

Your daughter won't eat. She's been this way for months, perhaps years. You've tried everything, but the situation remains the same. You dread mealtimes, and most days both of you end up in tears. Your daughter will not change, at least not until her own body requires more food, perhaps around five years old, or even in adolescence. Your three-year-old daughter can't come to you today, or next Monday, and say: "Mum, I've been thinking, and I've decided that starting today I will eat everything you put in front of me without a fight. This way you will know that I love you very much. I hope that this gesture will help improve our relationship." Your daughter is not able to reason in this way, and even if she were, she would never be able to keep her promise (since, as we've explained, she is physically unable to eat more than she needs without becoming ill).

The only hope for change, therefore, comes from you. You can tell your daughter: "Sweetheart, I've been thinking and I've decided that, starting today, I will not try to make you eat when you are not hungry, or to force you to eat foods that make you gag." You are able to keep your word (although of course, it will be hard).

Be sure to understand that what I propose here is not a new method to get your child to eat more. She will eat the same, more or less. What we are talking about is having her eat what she does eat happily, in a reasonable time frame, and not with two hours of crying, fighting and throwing up.

Let it also be understood that we are not talking about starving your child. The idea is not: "You are spoiled rotten, so I'm taking away the food, and now you'll know what it means to be hungry. When you are ready to eat, you will ask politely." Aside from being unfair, this would be dangerous, since you'd be engaging your daughter in a battle of wills, a battle that children often win. A couple of times I've seen (or rather, I've been told, years later) that the "don't make them eat" method failed. In both these cases it was used as a punishment (even without using those exact words, or even without uttering a word).

On the contrary, what we propose is to respect children's freedom and independence. The correct attitude is: "Darling, you're not hungry? Okay, then brush your teeth and go and play."

For most mothers who have spent years fighting about food, this change is a difficult one to make. All change is hard. And regarding food, it can be especially anxiety provoking. I've known mothers who had to go to another room to cry when they stopped trying to make their children eat. You are convinced that your daughter will not eat unless you make her. You think that she'll become anaemic or even "starve to death".

But your daughter isn't going to collapse on the spot and die from starvation. Before she became seriously ill, she would first have to lose weight, lots of weight. Remember how she lost weight at birth; many children lose 250 g (9 oz) in two days and are back up in less than a week, without any problems. If your daughter does not eat, she will lose weight, but she would have to lose a lot of weight before getting into real trouble. In the pictures we often see of malnourished children in Africa, these children have lost (or never gained) from 5 to 7 kg (11 to 15 lbs).

There is one very simple method that you can use to monitor your child's health to make sure she is not in any danger: a simple scale. While your child does not lose 1 kg (2.2 lbs), she is not in danger. I say 1 kg (perhaps less in smaller children, say, 10 percent of their weight) because smaller fluctuations in weight are totally normal and you would not have to worry about these. If you weighed your child before and after drinking a glass of water, she will have gained 250 g (9 oz) and if you weigh her after she uses the toilet, she may have lost almost half a kilo (about 1 lb). Less than one kilo (2.2.lbs) is irrelevant, and it's far removed from any danger.

Even if you are not convinced by the arguments in this book, and even if you still feel your daughter "won't eat unless we make her", I beg you to try this method, as an experiment. You have nothing to lose. You've been struggling for months, if not years, and you've tried everything. If you are right, by not making her eat she'll lose more than 1 kg (2.2 lbs) and lose it fast. (A newborn can lose 250 g (9 oz) in two days even while feeding; your daughter can easily lose more than one kilo 1 kg in less than one week, if she really does not eat.) If you are right, the experiment would have lasted a week or less and you can start making your child eat again and she'll recover her weight loss. You will have earned the right to tell all your neighbours that Dr. González's book was worthless.

But if I'm right, and by no longer making your child eat she does not lose even 1 kg, it would mean that she ate the same when forced to eat as she does when no longer forced. How much time do you spend trying to feed your child, breakfast, lunch, dinner and snacks? Many mothers spend more than four hours per day, four hours full of tears, screams and throwing up. Now your child might take around an hour a day to eat, and she won't even require your presence some of this time. Think of all the things you could do with your spare time: read books, write books, learn to play the piano – or simply, do much more enjoyable things with your daughter. Take that time to read stories together, draw, build, play and help her with her chores. If this experiment works, your life, your daughter's life, and your whole family's life will change.

In essence, the experiment is as follows:

1. Weigh your child on a scale.
2. Do not make your child eat.
3. Weigh your child again after a few days.
4. If your child hasn't lost 1 kg (2.2 lbs), go back to step 2.
5. If more than 1 kg has been lost, stop the experiment. Go back to doing whatever you want.

Some important points

The scale

A simple bathroom scale will do the trick, as long as it works well. You can also use a scale at a chemist's. Just be sure to use the same scale and have the child wear the same clothing (or no clothing at home). You'll save yourself some worry if you do your weighing at the same time of day, but it is not essential to do so. You can weigh your child as many times as you wish. I would weigh a child once a week, maximum, but if you are very worried, you can check the weight every day. Do not, under any circumstance, try to make your child eat unless he or she has lost at least 1 kg (2.2 lbs). Obviously, this experiment should be done when the child is healthy; not when she is sick with diarrhoea, a cold, or chicken pox, since it is easy for a child to lose 1 kg when sick, regardless of whether you try to make her eat or not.

Not making them eat

This implies that you won't force food by any means, not using any strategies, neither gently nor harshly. I know that you don't tie your child up to a chair and beat her. When I say "don't make her", I mean, don't do "the airplane" with the spoon, don't distract her with songs or television, don't promise her things if she finishes her food, don't threaten her with punishment. Do not beg or plead. Do not appeal to her love for you or to grandmother's approval. Do not compare her with her siblings, and don't speak of "good girls" and "bad girls". Do not make dessert conditional upon finishing her plate.

How not to force a child to eat

Let's suppose that today you're having macaroni, beef with potatoes, and banana as a dessert.

"Do you want macaroni?" "Yes." How many pieces of macaroni

does your child normally eat before starting to resist? Five? Well, put three on her plate. Three? Yes, not three tablespoons, not three lumps, three pieces of macaroni. Let her eat on her own, with her fingers or using a fork if she knows how to use it.

If she finishes those, you don't need to ask, "Do you want more macaroni, sweetie?" If she wants more, she'll ask. If after a few minutes she has not eaten them, you ask, "Oh, are you finished?" If she says she's finished, you take away the plate without giving her the evil eye and without reproach. If she says she's not finished, but does not eat, let her know politely that she needs to eat or that you will take away the plate. Take away the plate if she still has not shown signs of eating within a reasonable amount of time. The first few days, your daughter may be so used to taking two hours to eat that the change might surprise her; so be flexible and if she wants the plate back, go ahead and give it back.

If your daughter was used to being fed by an adult, try not to make this new method of asking her to feed herself feel like punishment or lack of attention. If she wants you to feed her, go ahead. If she is not eating, but doesn't want the plate to be taken away, you can offer to feed her: "Do you want help?" But do not feed your child unless she has asked for or accepted help, and stop as soon as she no longer wants more.

It may also be that she is not interested in even trying the macaroni. Without reaction, without a change in your tone of voice, you offer the second item.

Whether she ate five pieces of macaroni or none, you start over with the next item: ask if she wants any, put less on her plate than what you think she'll happily eat. Now remember that many two- or three-year-olds eat a portion of beef about the size of a postage stamp, and that is if they are very hungry. If she only wants potatoes, go ahead and give her only potatoes.

The example I've used includes two food items because many families cook this way. But some families only prepare one dish, and that is just fine. I am in no way suggesting you should prepare two different items.

When she no longer wants more of the second item, it's time for dessert. Do not try to bribe her with dessert ("If you finish all your meat, you can have chocolate ice cream") and don't pressure her ("We can't have ice cream until you finish your meat") and definitely do not make fun of her ("Well, here is dessert, but if you really were that hungry, you could have eaten more meat"). Also, do not blame her ("Here I am, slaving over a hot stove to make a nice dinner, but the little princess here would rather eat yogurt"). If she does not want dessert either, let her go and play.

Keep in mind that the size of the packaging of commercial products like yogurt is set with adults in mind. When you eat a yogurt, you eat one, not half a dozen. You should not expect your daughter at three years old to eat the same amount. Maybe she does eat it, and it's not a problem (of course, that will be her whole dinner). But if she's eaten other things first, she will probably eat about one-fourth of the yogurt. It is not reasonable to expect her to finish it all. And don't come back and tell me, "Well, my parents always fed me two", because that would be a lie.

In the same manner, when you eat a banana, an orange, or an apple, you probably only eat one piece. No one takes a bunch of bananas and starts eating them as if they were grapes. It is not reasonable to expect your daughter to eat a whole banana, or a whole apple, unless that is the only thing she's eating.

Do not use the punishment: "Well, now I'm putting away the macaroni and until you eat them, cold and dry or however, you won't get anything else." At the next meal, give her what you are going to give everyone else. (Of course, many households will eat leftovers for another meal. Do this if that is what you normally do, but not to punish.)

Let's suppose your daughter eats nothing for breakfast, nothing for lunch, nothing for a snack, nothing for dinner. Are you concerned about what may happen? Weigh her then. If she has not lost 1 kg (2.2 lbs) yet, keep on going. This is a good time to stop and think about how the experiment is going. Are you sure that other family members are not trying to make your child eat? Are you sure that you are not using prodding, insinuation, or other psychological pressures instead of physical force?

It is unlikely that your daughter will really go all day without eating. It is almost guaranteed that she will eat

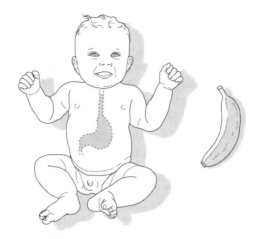

A nine-month-old and a banana drawn to scale.
Where can the banana go?

something, and it will usually be very close to what she was eating before the experiment. Were you to weigh her the next day, she probably would not have lost or gained anything.

It is also possible that, due to her new-found freedom, she may not eat at all at mealtime and that after a couple of hours she may get hungry. You can feed her then, as long as it's a "healthy" snack. You can choose from the food she previously declined (if that's what she wants, not as a punishment), or any other food that you have on hand: a banana, a yogurt, or a sandwich. Try to avoid two mistakes: first, to offer treats instead of healthful foods. Second, to become a short-order cook. It's one thing to not force your child to eat and another to spend an extra hour in the kitchen because the precious darling wanted spaghetti, not macaroni. Any family member, no matter their age, who does not like what is for dinner does not have to eat what has been prepared. But they will have to make do with whatever they can grab (at least until they learn to cook). Every privilege also brings with it responsibility. The privilege of cooking what you want for dinner means you have to put up with the protests of the members of the family who wanted something else. In order to avoid having to cook two meals and to avoid fighting, many parents end up only cooking meals they know their children will like. Pasta, rice, and French fries become staples in households with young children.

At this point, you may be concerned about manners. I was taught as a youngster that food is not meant to be thrown, and it seems reasonable to expect children to finish what they asked for, but not what others tried to force on them. Also, small children can make a mistake and ask for more than they can eat. They will get better at this as time goes by. It is also common among adults to eat all that is set in front of you, even if you don't like it. When we eat at a friend's house, we pretend we like things we don't and eat them anyway (although many adults have no problem leaving a plateful at a restaurant). But, did we do this at five? In some families it is expected that no one leave the table until everyone finishes eating. If any of these rules of etiquette seem important to you, by all means, teach them to your daughter . . . but not today. Today you are trying to solve a serious problem. There will be lots of time later to teach, with love and patience, all about good manners. You cannot expect a three-year-old to behave like an adult.

So what can you do in the meantime so you're not throwing away leftover food? Well, to begin with, don't put so much food on the plate. Your child will not eat the same every day, of course, but if you put an adequate amount on the plate, there should be only a few teaspoonfuls left on his plate every once in a while. And if you don't want to throw this away, you can eat it yourself. But if every day there is half a plateful of food left over, then you are giving your child twice as much as what he needs. You are the one wasting the food by insisting on serving your child a much larger portion than what you know he can eat.

But does this really work?

The story of Adriana and her son, Juan, is a perfect example of the painful depths that a family can reach when they are told they must make their child eat, and how easily this problem can be solved, with a little common sense.

From the start Adriana had many obstacles in trying to breastfeed her son: the nurses refused to bring her the baby until six hours after the birth, in spite of her requests. And later they told her, "If he is not breastfeeding, he needs food", and proceeded to bottle-feed him.

The story is so typical: bottles, jaundice, weight loss, sore nipples . . .

I gave up breastfeeding after both the doctor and the nurse laughed at my attempts.

But bottle-feeding was not so easy. Juan would not drink the "proper" amount and was not following the growth curve (see pages 33–6). He was sent to several doctors and tried every kind of formula (including pre-digested, hypoallergenic kinds). He was admitted into the hospital for two gastric scopes, allergy testing, contrast testing and lab tests.

They finally found a pyloric mass that seemed to be partially obstructing the outlet of his stomach. Although they were not quite sure that this was the reason for our problems, it was all that they could find. At least it was something at last.

After this we started with constipation, suppositories, laxatives, enemas. Next the doctors started him on solids early, to see if that would help. Baby food jars, powdered baby food, and a whole lot of food that all went to waste.

Our son has grown very slowly, he throws up every day, and every day we scold, threaten, bribe, sing, go out to the porch, spank, get toys, make faces, tell stories, etc.

At two years and nine months, Juan weighed 12 kg (26 lbs 7 oz). He would throw up, had "behaviour issues", had been to a psychologist, and was still going to the gastroenterologist. It was at this time that his mother read the first edition of this book:

Our life has completely changed, he eats more than he used to. At first he was confused, as if mystified that we were not making him finish his plate. He seemed to think we were crazy or something. Now he eats more, and eats better. He even asks to eat at times other than mealtime. The change is like night and day, ever since the first day we started to apply this . . .

His behaviour has also improved although there is much to be done yet. So much damage to repair. Right now he's going through a difficult stage, since he seems to be a little jealous of his baby sister. But I suppose that is to be expected. One thing that has helped him is that every day I express some of my milk (70 to 90 ml or 2.5 to 3 oz) for him and I give it to him in a cup. He sees me expressing this milk for him, and knows it's the same milk that his sister gets, and I think that reassures him. I have also noticed that since I am giving him my milk he has not had one cold, and it's been more than one month . . .

I am enraged that my family and especially my son had to go through all this; all while he was totally healthy and normal.

Of course, reading this book does not always work so well, you can ask Aurora who writes:

Just as I finished reading this book, my daughter quit eating. She's still happy as a clam.

I swear that it was not my book's fault. What happened is that Aurora read the book just as her daughter turned twelve months, and, as we've explained, a decrease in appetite seems to occur at that age.

Part III
How to avoid the problem in the first place

Chapter 6
Breastfeeding without conflict

Clear advice

As is true of most other things, conflicts with children surrounding food are much easier to prevent than to treat. The title and content of this book will very seldom attract the attention of pregnant couples, or of the parents of young babies who are still not eating solids. The majority of my readers will be parents who are desperate because it's been several months and their child "won't eat".

But I don't lose heart. Perhaps you are pregnant, or your child is still young, and this book has been loaned or recommended to you by a friend or sister-in-law who has been through this. Or you might be thinking about having another child and you'd like nothing more than to avoid eating problems a second time.

Therefore, this section contains some tips on how to feed your child in order to avoid conflicts.

I cannot state this any more clearly:

> **Do not force your child to eat.**
> **Never make him eat, in any way,**
> **under any circumstance, for any reason.**

This advice only takes three lines and you might think it's not worth the price you paid for this book. So I will elaborate further.

But everything else is fluff and, if at any moment you are lost in my explanations and you need to return to the basics, come back to these three lines.

Trust your child

Let's go back to the beginning. After nine long months of waiting, you finally have your baby in your arms. Stop! Although there will be many who will try to tell you otherwise, that is the best place for your baby.

To avoid problems from the start, the main thing is to trust your child. Your child knows if he is hungry. The clock does not. Most children will nurse between eight and twelve times a day, at irregular intervals. They usually take fifteen to twenty minutes per breast in the early weeks, while they are learning, but at around two to four months, they sometimes nurse very quickly, and are finished in five to seven minutes or even less. This is what most of them do, but there is always one that beats the record, by nursing for a longer or shorter time. If you breastfeed when he asks, and let him nurse as long as he wants, your child will always receive the milk he needs.

Offer the breast on demand

We have explained earlier why you should breastfeed on demand (see chapters 2 and 4). You will remember that babies do not usually have a regular schedule, because it is precisely this variation in schedule that allows them to modify the composition of the milk to adapt it to their needs.

It is said that our civilization is afraid of true freedom; that may explain why so many people cannot accept breastfeeding on demand and therefore try to impose limits. The saddest part is that sometimes these limits are imposed so subtly that it seems as though we are talking about the same thing, but it is not the same. For example, read these common misconceptions:

First misconception: *"Offer the breast on demand, that is, not earlier than two-and-a-half hours and no later than four."*

This is not demand feeding. It is a flexible schedule and, although it is more or less in the ballpark, it is not demand feeding. Why not nurse before two-and-a-half hours? Has it never happened to you that right after a meal you meet a friend and you go and have coffee? Or do you tell your friend: "You go ahead and have some coffee, I'll keep you company. I just ate and I'm not due to eat again until five o'clock"?

Second misconception: *"In the first few weeks it is advisable to feed on demand; after a while your child will settle into his own pattern."*

Not all children find a pattern. And among those who do settle into a routine, very few follow it with the military rigour that this phrase seems to imply (every two hours, or every three, or every four). It is much more likely that the chosen rhythm will be like the "cha-cha-cha": several nursings clumped together, others more clearly spaced, and one longer pause.[25] Breastfeeding patterns, when they happen, tend to be followed from one day to the next. If Laura usually nurses frequently during the morning and then sleeps a long time in the afternoon, it is likely that she will repeat this pattern tomorrow. But she may also surprise you, and that is the beauty of having children. They are people, not robots.

Third misconception: *"Try to stretch the time between feeds."*

This is also not demand feeding. Why are people so obsessed with lengthening the time between feeds? Your baby wants to nurse and you want to feed him, why should anyone have anything to say about this? Should you also try to stretch the time between kisses? How would you like it if your time between Sunday and Sunday got "stretched"? Or between payday and payday, or vacation and vacation? Perhaps our bosses would be happy with a Sunday every ten days, paying us every forty-three days and giving us two weeks vacation every year-and-a-half, but they don't even think to propose this. Well then, your baby would be just as indignant if he could speak and he were to find out that someone wished to "stretch the time between feeds". (For more information on the disadvantages of "stretching the time between feeds" see the FAQ "Is it bad to eat between meals?" on page 156.)

Crisis at three months of age

Around two to three months, some babies get so good at nursing that they are able to get what they need in five or seven minutes, sometimes even in three minutes or less. If no one has told the mother about this, if all she's heard is "ten minutes", she's going to think her baby is not nursing enough, just like Encarna:

> I have a four-month-old daughter. My problem is that I don't know if she's eating enough. She only spends three or four minutes on the breast and I'm afraid she's not getting enough milk. When she was two months old, she would eat ten minutes on the first side and five minutes on the other side and was gaining weight quickly; now she seems to be falling short on the growth curve. I have also noted that my breasts are not as full as before; they used to leak.
>
> What is puzzling is that, during the first few minutes she swallows a lot and very fast, then she starts coming on and off the breast, and she won't sit still. I have to alternate sides and try different positions to get her to nurse for at least ten minutes. I wonder if she is doing this because she's still hungry or what.
>
> Something else is that she is eating more frequently now, especially at night. She was sleeping five to six hours at a time, now she only sleeps for three or occasionally four hours.
>
> The doctor has told me I can start giving her formula in a bottle. I've tried and she doesn't want it, even if someone else offers the bottle.

This mother's story illustrates all the aspects of this "crisis at three months":

1. A baby who was nursing for ten minutes or more is now finished in five minutes or less.
2. Breasts that once felt heavy or full are now soft.
3. Milk no longer leaks.
4. Baby's weight slows down.

All this is absolutely normal. Breast fullness in the first few weeks has little to do with the amount of milk and is more accurately a temporary inflammation that happens at the beginning of lactation. Engorgement and leaking are "start up" problems that disappear when breastfeeding is comfortably established.

And the slower weight gain, of course, is to be expected. Babies gain less and less in each subsequent month. That is why growth curves are curves. Otherwise they would be straight lines. Between one and two months, breastfed baby girls typically gain between 500 g and 1.5 kg (1 lb 2 oz to 3 lbs 5 oz) with the average being slightly over 1,000 g (2 lbs 3 oz). We have excluded the first month since there is usually some weight loss and gain, which makes the amounts too variable. If babies were to keep gaining at this pace, in one year they would gain 6 to 18 kg (13 to 40 lbs) with an average of over 12 kg (26 lbs). Actually, during the first year of life, baby girls gain between 4.5 kg and 7 kg (10 to 15 lbs) with the mean being 6 kg (13 lbs). In other words, even a baby girl who gained 500 g (1 lb 2 oz) in her first month (some might think that is too low, but it is really normal) will eventually gain even less. All the weights given are approximate and rounded. Male babies often gain a little more than girls.

Of course Encarna's baby did not want the bottle; she wasn't hungry. Unfortunately not all babies show this restraint and sometimes, especially if we insist, they will take a bottle even if they are not hungry. Don't try this just to see if it works!

Had someone taken the time to explain to Encarna that this was about to happen, she would not have worried at all. But the change took her by surprise.

Surprise and all, had Encarna been confident and sure of her ability to breastfeed, she would not have worried. Because the most logical explanation for all these changes is: "I have so much milk that my daughter gets full in only three minutes." But the fear of failure in breastfeeding is so great in our society, that no matter what is going on, the mother will always think (or will be told) she does not have enough milk.

This mother is also worried because of another modern myth: that children, as time goes by, learn to sleep longer. In reality, children spend more time awake. It is true that someday they will sleep more hours in a row and they may start sleeping through the night somewhere around three or four years of age. But hardly at four months. Between birth and four months the change you are most likely to observe in your child is that he will sleep less. Most babies nurse several times each night during the first years (which is always much easier than giving bottles late at night, especially if the baby is in bed with you).

This mother has already started to force her daughter to eat. It's all downhill from here. It is easy to predict that unless mother decides to make a radical change, the introduction of solid foods will be a struggle.

What can I do to increase milk production?

Why on earth do you want to have more milk? Are you thinking about opening a dairy business?

The concern mothers have about adequate milk production is ancient: centuries ago, when everyone breastfed, prayers were directed to saints and virgins who "specialized" in good, abundant milk, and mothers used herbs and concoctions with solid reputations.

Perhaps this fear stems from ignorance. People believed that the amount of milk depended on the mother – there were mothers who made lots of milk and others who made little; mothers who made good milk and others who made bad milk.

In most cases, the amount of milk does not depend on the

mother, but on the baby. There are babies who nurse a lot and babies who don't and the amount of milk will always be exactly as much as the baby takes out.

Exactly? Yes. Milk production is regulated minute-by-minute by the amount of milk your baby has taken at the previous feeding. If the baby was very hungry and quickly emptied the breast, then the milk will be produced at great speed. If, however, the child was not too interested and left the breast half full, then the milk will be made more slowly. This has been demonstrated through careful calculations measuring the increase in volume available in the breast between feedings.[26]

For the mother to have insufficient milk, that is, less than what her baby needs, one of the following conditions must be present:

1. A baby who does **not nurse enough** (for example, if baby is sick or full of sugar water or tea or if baby has been given bottles).
2. A baby who **nurses, but incorrectly** (for example, if baby places his tongue incorrectly because he has gotten used to pacifiers and bottles, or if he is weak because of losing too much weight, or because of a neurological problem, or a tongue-tie that stops him from moving his tongue freely).
3. A baby who is **not allowed to nurse**, because people want to feed him according to a schedule, or to entertain him with a pacifier when he shows hunger cues.

Other than these three instances (or a few other situations that may happen very rarely), almost all mothers will have exactly the amount of milk that their baby needs.

Therefore, when asked: "What can I do to increase my milk?" the first thing would be to establish if there is really a problem (if the child is losing weight or gaining very slowly). If this is so, it will be a matter of figuring out which of the three scenarios above is involved (or it may be all three) and then fixing it. If the baby is sick, we need to find out what his problem is and treat it. If he is so weak he can't nurse, then express milk and feed him using another method. If he was getting water or a pacifier, stop giving those. If he was getting bottles, stop those, too. (This will have to be done gradually, if he has been getting lots of them.) If positioning was the problem, fix it so that he can learn. A breastfeeding support group will be helpful.*

However there are many, many instances in which the mother believes (erroneously), for one reason or another, that she does not have enough milk.

Some of the false "symptoms" of insufficient milk are:

- The baby cries.
- The baby does not cry.
- The baby wants to be fed more frequently than every three hours.
- It's been three hours and the baby is not asking to feed.
- The baby takes more than ten minutes to nurse.
- The baby nurses in five minutes and doesn't want any more.
- The baby nurses at night.
- The baby doesn't nurse at night.
- My mother didn't have milk either.
- My mother had lots of milk.
- My breasts are too full.
- My breasts are too empty.
- My breasts are too small.
- My breasts are too large.
- I don't have a nipple.
- I have three nipples. (Did you laugh? Many mothers tell me in all seriousness that they "don't have a nipple". I assure you it is much more common to have three nipples than none.)

When worried about any of these symptoms, the mother decides to do something to increase her milk. If she decides to do something useless but harmless, like eating almonds or lighting a candle to Saint Anthony, probably nothing bad will happen and it may even be possible that her faith may make her believe that her milk has increased, and everyone will be happy. But sometimes

---

* For example see www.breastfeedingnetwork.org.uk, www.laleche.org.uk, www.abm.me.uk, www.nct.org.uk, www.thebabycafe.org

the mother tries something that does work, or at least has the potential of working. In those cases, the advice from people who know something about human lactation can do more harm than the advice from people who know nothing, especially in a case where the mother's milk supply is not a problem at all.

Elena's story shows us the depth of anguish that can be provoked when you combine the ten-minute rule, anxiety about weight gain and some seemingly reasonable yet irrelevant advice, since there was no problem to fix in the first place:

My son is three months and ten days old. He weighs only 5.640 kg (12 lbs 7 oz). When he was born he weighed 3.120 kg (6 lbs 14 oz) and he lost in the first few days to 2.760 kg (6 lbs 1 oz). The main problem is that he never wants to nurse. At first I would feed him every three hours, but he always nursed only a little. The doctor suggested I nurse him every two hours, and since things did not improve, it was suggested that I put him to the breast all the time. Things have not improved at all and in fact are worse. The baby only nurses well at night, and during the day when he is half asleep. I've done everything I've been told: from pumping some milk before offering the breast so he can get "high calorie" milk, to eliminating all dairy from my diet. Nothing has worked and I'm going crazy. We've even tried giving him the bottle and he doesn't want it. The doctor says he is healthy (having done several lab tests) and normal, but this situation is very distressing for me. I live in constant anguish, worried if he'll eat at the next feeding or not, always watching to see when he goes to sleep so I can put him on the breast and waiting to see if by chance he happens to swallow. I can't go out or do anything in case the baby decides to nurse. I am also very worried because his weight is under the mean.

This baby's weight falls in the 7th percentile; that is, seven out of 100 healthy babies his age will weigh less. That would be 52,500 out of the 750,000 babies born in the UK each year. How are the mothers of those other 52,500 children managing? This weight is totally normal.

However, the problem was not the weight, but the fact that this baby "nurses very little". What that means here is that (since this baby was breastfeeding and we don't know how much he was really taking) the baby was nursing very quickly. How much pain would have been avoided if this mother would have known that some babies nurse very quickly and others nurse slower and that it is not necessary to watch the clock. How much better would it have been if the first time this mother said "my baby eats so little", someone had said: "Of course! He is so smart that he's figured out how to nurse efficiently and quickly." Instead she was told that there was a problem, this baby was not nursing long enough ... and she was given advice to nurse him more. Advice naturally destined for failure since the baby did not need to nurse more, and therefore could not.

In four short months, the situation has deteriorated to the point that the baby only nurses while asleep. A psychologist could have spoken about food aversions that keep him from nursing while awake. Perhaps he would explain about the "good breast/bad breast". But we don't need to look at psychological abstractions to become aware that, if the baby has already nursed while asleep and has taken all he needed (which is evident since he keeps growing normally), it is impossible to add more nursings while he is awake. He would be eating twice as much as he needs. He would burst.

This baby will not be able to nurse when he is awake as long as his mother continues to breastfeed him in his sleep. And he is only four months old, has yet to taste solids and experience the normal appetite loss at one year. If something doesn't change, the situation in this family may become desperate.

How does the child see this situation? Of course, he doesn't understand what is going on. He does not know he's supposed to nurse for ten minutes and that his weight is in the 7th percentile. He was fine, nursing as he wished, when all of a sudden strange things started taking place. He was getting woken up to nurse much more frequently and as best he could he tried to be accommodating, making the feedings shorter, of course. Sometimes someone had removed the skim milk at the beginning of the feeding and from the first suck he was getting cream, full of fat and calories. As is to be expected, these feedings were even shorter. Naturally, he did not want to try the bottle. ("But I've already nursed eight times today!") Each time he responded in a logical manner, unable to understand his mother and those who would counsel her. A few weeks ago he started having some strange "nightmares". He dreams that a breast is introduced into his mouth and that his stomach gets full of milk. The strangest thing is how real this dream seems, he even wakes up stuffed full and unable to nurse during the day.

His mother seems more worried with each passing day; he sees her crying sometimes and that frightens him. If he could talk, he would most likely say the same thing that his mother says to us: "She's driving me crazy." And were he able to understand what is happening, he would certainly make an effort to nurse more slowly and stay the required ten minutes on the breast. (Drinking the same amount, of course, no point getting indigestion.) That way everyone would be happy. But he does not understand what is happening and cannot make a goodwill gesture. Only his mother can change; otherwise the problem will remain for months or even years.

Why your baby won't take a bottle

We have a four-and-a-half-month old daughter. She weighs 5.950 kg (13 lbs 2 oz). Up till now she has been fully breastfed, but we think we may have to start supplementing. The problem is that she rejects the bottle. We have tried to give her a bottle before nursing, as well as after. Either way she rejects it.

I never did find out why these parents felt they had to supplement their daughter. It is obvious that the baby didn't know either. So, please tell me, what else does a baby need to do to let people know that he does not need or want a bottle?

Little children, especially in their first two months are so naïve that sometimes they let themselves be fooled into taking a bottle, even if they are not hungry. But older babies often resist tooth and nail – enough is enough!

Why your baby does not seem interested in other foods

Generally speaking, bottle-fed infants accept solids better than breastfed babies. This is probably because human milk contains all the nutrients and vitamins that your baby needs, while formula does not. Are you surprised? Every few years, formula manufacturers bombard us with publicity highlighting some new ingredient that they have just added to their product in order to make it "more like mother's milk". In a few short years we've seen taurine, nucleotides, long-chain polyunsaturated fatty acids, selenium . . . The milk we were given as babies had none of those things. Since they keep researching, we can expect more additions in years to come. The mother's milk that you make every day has all the ingredients that will be in formula ten, fifty, and five hundred years from now.

With our current knowledge, the most sensible thing to do is to start offering other foods at six months. Some children eat happily and probably do need them. But we say, "offer" not "stuff". The child is free to eat or not. Many breastfed babies do not want anything to do with other foods until eight or ten months, sometimes longer. They are healthy and happy, their weight and height are normal, and they are hitting all the developmental milestones. They have all they need with the breast and therefore want nothing else.

This produces much anxiety in the mothers of these breastfed babies between six and twelve months. Their children barely peck at food (a bite of banana here, a breadcrumb there, one noodle over there) other than the breast. You can always hear a not-so-helpful remark: "Your Laura doesn't eat yet? Well you should see my Jessica, she just loves her mixed cereal with milk."

He who laughs last, laughs best. Breastfed babies may take longer to accept other foods, but when they do start eating, they often bypass any commercial baby foods or strained preparations and throw themselves at their mother's plate. At the beginning of the second year, the breastfed baby will typically eat lentils with sausage, potato omelette, and ham sandwiches, all by the spoonful, and bite full and all by their own hand.

Others, like Julia's son, do things backwards; they accept baby food for a while and then seem to change their mind.

What do you do if a child, at fifteen months, after eating normally since he was six months old, now does not want to eat? His only thought is to nurse. When he turned ten months old he would only take the breast to go to sleep, but once he turned a year, he started to reject food and now only wants to breastfeed.

What should be done? Nothing. If you leave him well enough alone, in a few weeks or months the baby will once again be interested in other food. If instead you try to make him eat other foods, or try to withhold breastfeeding, no doubt he will also eat other other foods someday (I assure you he will not still be just breastfeeding when he is twenty), but probably it will take longer and be much harder on both of you

Chapter 7
Bottle-feeding without conflict

Bottles are also offered on demand

For a time, when the idea of demand feeding for breastfed infants started to become fashionable, many people reasoned that this was recommended because: "Human milk is so digestible and gastric emptying time for human milk is so much shorter." They believed that bottle-fed babies must be fed on a schedule to avoid intestinal difficulties, because formula is harder to digest.

The thing is no one knows what these intestinal difficulties might be. The current recommendations, starting with those given by ESPGAN (1982), state that the bottle, just like the breast, should be given on demand, both in time and in quantity.[18]

How many mothers have been forced to stop breastfeeding because their baby "was not gaining enough", only to find that he won't finish the bottles and that he gains even less weight after weaning from the breast!

If your baby finishes 120 ml (4 oz) easily, then give him 150 ml (5 oz). But if he always leaves 30 ml (1 oz), then make the next bottle with 90 ml (3 oz) – the formula isn't free, you know. If he is hungry before three hours have elapsed, then give him another bottle. And if one day he sleeps for five hours, then go ahead and take a nap, since this is not something that happens every day.

Why your child won't finish the bottle

Our son is two-and-a-half months. He was 2.950 kg (6 lbs 8 oz) at birth and is now 5.840 kg (12 lbs 14 oz). In the past two weeks he has gained 100 and 80 g (3.5 and 2.8 oz). I would not be so worried about this except that he does not finish his bottles. He is still only drinking 120 ml (4 oz) at a time, if we're lucky.

Rosana's concern deserves an additional comment. She says that, if her son were finishing the bottles, she would not worry about his weight. When I explain to mothers that their child's weight is normal, just like Rosana's baby's, I have heard hundreds of times: "I don't want him to be fat, all I want is for him to eat more." But how is it possible to eat more and not gain more? Unless the child had a parasite!

Many children do not finish their bottle. The amount of milk recommended on the can for a certain age, or the amount recommended by your doctor, will always be on the high side. It must be on the high side. Not all children need the same amount of milk. If the experts conclude that children need between 120 ml (4 oz) and 160 ml (5.5 oz) of milk, they are not going to instruct parents to only give 120 ml, because this would not be enough for almost all children. Nor will they recommend the average, 140 ml, because this would be too little for half of the children. To leave a child hungry is obviously more dangerous than to have a little milk left in the bottle, so they should say at least 160 ml. Of course, these calculations are based on the most common cases and the most common children. So, what if some need more, or we've been mistaken in our calculations? Should we put 165 ml (5.5 oz) on the can just in case? But since formula is prepared using one scoop per 30 ml (1 oz) of water, and the mother will have a hard time measuring exactly half of that, we round up the amount to 180 ml (6 oz). The result is that no child goes hungry, but many leave some milk in their bottle. If no one told the mother that the child might not finish the bottle, and that this is normal, she might try to force her baby to take all 180 ml, when her baby was one of those who only needed 120 ml (4 oz).

So the battle ensues.

Many doctors believe that one of the great advantages of breastfeeding is that you cannot see how much a baby has left. And the proposal to make bottles out of aluminium so that the mother can't see if they are empty is an old joke in our profession.

Chapter 8
Solid foods: a touchy subject

The struggles between mother and child around breastfeeding or bottles can be awful; but they are mercifully infrequent. The introduction of solids is a new opportunity for danger, and we must tread this path very carefully.

By the way, when mentioning "solids" we do not only refer to those baby foods that are given with a spoon. As explained earlier (see "Recommendations from ESPGAN" on page 71), we will use this term to refer to anything other than human milk or formula, be it to liquids, such as tea, or to solids, such as a cracker.

Many mothers find themselves overwhelmed by the amount of rules, big ones, little ones, and medium ones surrounding infant feeding. They receive advice from the doctor and nurses, recommendations many times much more complex and detailed than those from top experts, advice from family and friends, as well as old wives' tales that warn about avoiding "harsh foods" and "incompatible" ones.

Unable to follow all the rules at the same time, frequently the mother opts for rejecting everything and doing whatever she pleases. The risk is that she might bypass the directives that really are important. To avoid this problem, I will differentiate clearly between those topics over which there is some degree of a consensus regarding their importance (based on a combination of international norms as discussed in chapter 4's feeding guides on page 71), and those pieces of advice that seem helpful to me, though others may have their own opinion.

When revising this book I realised I had included too many rules. In retrospect, some of these aren't as important as I had suggested. They were based on expert opinion rather than on any scientific studies, and it seems the experts have since changed their minds.

Some important points

It is important to keep in mind the following points, although they should not be taken as dogma:

1. Never force a child to eat.
2. Breastfeed exclusively for six months (no baby food, juice, water, teas, etc.).
3. Starting at six months, offer (without forcing) other foods, and always after breastfeeding. Non-breastfed children should be offered at least 500 ml (17 oz) of formula per day.
4. At first, don't offer too many new foods together, and start with small amounts.
5. Give gluten-containing foods (wheat, oats, barley, or rye) with caution.
6. When cooking foods for babies, drain well, to avoid filling baby up with water.
7. There is no hurry to introduce highly allergenic foods (especially dairy, eggs, fish, soy, peanuts, and any food that other members of the family may be allergic to).
8. Do not add salt or sugar to foods.
9. Keep breastfeeding for two years or beyond.

Sometimes you can give a baby food before six months (but never before four): when mother has to work, for example. Or when the child clearly is asking to be fed by trying to grab food and putting it in his mouth.

"To offer", means that if he wants to eat, he eats, and if not, he doesn't. Many children don't want anything but the breast until eight or ten months, sometimes longer.

Solids are offered after breastfeeding, not before, and certainly not in place of breastfeeding. Only then can you make sure your child will drink the milk he needs. It is believed that between six and twelve months, babies need about 500 ml (17 oz) of milk per day. Of course this is an average amount, many children drink more and others are fine with less. A child who drinks from a bottle can easily get this amount by drinking two 250 ml (9 oz) bottles a day. It is not reasonable, however, to expect a breastfed baby to nurse 250 ml every twelve hours; the mother's breasts would be uncomfortably full. It makes much more sense for breastfed babies to nurse 100 ml (3.3 oz) five times a day, or 70 ml (2.3 oz) seven times a day. Of course you don't know (nor did you know before starting solids) how much milk your baby is drinking; but if you breastfeed before offering solids, you can rest assured he is getting what he needs.

Step by step. In previous editions I gave importance to some AAP advice from 1980 about introducing new foods one by one at intervals of at least a week, in order to see whether any of them disagreed with the baby. In fact no scientific research has been carried out that shows this is necessary, appropriate or useful. It simply seemed logical and reasonable. However, it is a rule that can easily turn into an obsession when it comes to allowing our children to experiment: "This morning I gave him some banana, and this afternoon he tried to take some bread, what do I do? He shouldn't be having bread for another week!" I still don't think it is a good idea when he is six months and a day old to give him too many different foods at once, but I wouldn't worry about his trying two or three new foods in the same day.

Gluten. The first edition of this book recommended offering gluten at eight months, but even then I warned that it was debatable. Gluten has indeed been debated in the scientific community. The concern is that, in people with a genetic predisposition, gluten triggers a very severe ailment: celiac disease. Recent studies in Scandinavia,[25,26] confirm that breastfeeding reduced the risk of celiac disease, but that the main protective factor was not the late introduction of gluten as was previously thought, but the gradual introduction of gluten while the child was still breastfeeding.

In practical terms what this means is that it is best to have the child continue to breastfeed for at least one month (and more is better) after introducing gluten, and that for the first month or two, it is best to only offer small amounts of gluten. If you plan to wean your child at seven or eight months, it is better that their first food contains gluten. And if you decide to breastfeed for longer, is it best to introduce glutens later? This isn't completely clear, although in some studies introducing gluten after seven months is associated with a slightly higher risk of celiac disease, which is why the ESPGHAN (2008)[29] recommends introducing it before seven months.

So how do you go about offering only small amounts of gluten? If you give your baby commercial cereal, you could prepare a gluten-free cereal and add half a teaspoon of gluten-containing cereal. Carry on adding half or one teaspoon of gluten to the babyfood for one or two months; after that you can increase the amount of cereals containing gluten. If you make your own baby food, you can have the baby's main dish without gluten (for example, cooked rice), but let him have a small piece of bread each day, or a couple of pieces of macaroni, but not more. After one or two months you can increase the amount of gluten cereal, bread, or pasta.

Remember, biscuits or cookies do contain gluten, since they are usually made from wheat flour. I remember, as a young paediatrician, when we recommended introducing gluten at nine months, and how annoyed we were with grandmothers who gave the baby a biscuit with his pureed fruit "to make it more nourishing". "What's the point", we railed, "of telling mothers to give their children gluten-free cereals, if grandmothers insist on giving the child biscuits?" Well, it turns out those grandmothers were probably right, and giving babies those tiny amounts of gluten at six months prevented some of them from getting celiac disease. A new lesson in humility.

Allergenic foods. In 1982 the ESPGAN advised not introducing the most allergenic foods as a general rule until six months, and not until twelve months in children who had a family history of allergies. In the year 2000, advice from the American Academy of Paediatrics (AAP)[30] was even more zealous: for children with a family history of allergies, they recommended not introducing cow's milk or its derivatives, until one year; eggs, not until two years; fish and dried fruits, not until three years. However the trend is changing. That advice was based on expert opinion, and some rather inconclusive research. Subsequent studies have also proved inconclusive. Based on the available data, both the ESPGHAN[31] and the AAP[32] currently consider that delaying the introduction of certain foods has little effect on the risk of allergy.

For babies who are bottle-fed, it is best to keep them on infant formula until one year, and to avoid giving them yogurt, custard or cow's milk. But be careful: "adapted milk" isn't the same as "products prepared with adapted milk". If you wanted, you could make custard, ice cream, café au lait or yogurt using adapted milk. So, before one year make sure you only give them proper adapted milk, not some other product containing adapted milk. After one year they can take cow's milk. It is best to give only breastmilk to babies who are breastfeeding until they reach a year old. There is no need to mix milk into their babyfood (in fact it isn't a good idea). Babies who are breastfeeding don't take cereal mixed with milk: first they breastfeed, then they take cereal on its own (that is, milk-free cereal prepared with water), and the two are mixed up in the baby's stomach (the child doesn't need shaking, of course!).

Now then, it is one thing to give him a whole helping of non-adapted milk, or yogurt or custard, and quite another to let him try small amounts of food containing some milk (for example a piece of croquette, or the filling from a cannelloni). When a baby is bottle-fed without any problem, we already know he isn't allergic to cow's milk, and therefore it doesn't matter if he has small amounts of cow's milk contained in other foods. Also, for babies who are breastfeeding, it is unlikely to be a problem if they consume small amounts of other foods containing cow's milk before one year old. However, in families with a history of allergies, and even though there is no research to back this up, I still think it is wise to wait until the baby is one year old, because cow's milk (including from the bottle) is the most common cause of allergies in children.

Years ago, egg yolk was introduced first, followed by egg whites. This was done for two reasons: the egg white is most allergenic, and yolks are high in iron so it seemed sensible to offer the yolk first. However, new scientific data has disproved these two arguments. Although the yolk is not allergenic, it is impossible to totally separate it from the white, not even in a hard-boiled egg. Yolks will always have some egg white and may trigger a severe reaction in a person allergic to eggs. On the other hand, although the yolk is high in iron, it also contains factors that inhibit its absorption,[2] so it's not the great source of iron that it was once hailed to be. In conclusion, it's not worth the effort to try to separate whites from yolks.

Sugar and salt. No sugar and no salt? Nope. Sugar and salt consumption in adults is already too high these days; the longer a baby can get along without them, the better. Honey is also not good since it can carry botulism spores and in the United States it is recommended that honey not be given to children younger than twelve months. Brown sugar, molasses, and rice sugar are all still sugar.

Moreover, adding sugar and salt to a child's food is usually another ruse to make him eat; if you put enough sugar on his fruit or in his yogurt and smother his vegetables with salt he will eat it all up. We have already said that children show a natural preference toward sweet and salty foods. But in nature you cannot find pure salt or sugar; the modern ability to add these to foods allows for the manipulation of appetite control and makes our children eat more than they should. This is one reason why, even if they don't promote cavities, it is also not good to add artificial sweeteners to baby foods. Remember, the problem is not the few teaspoons of sugar he might ingest today, but the lifetime of sugar that he will ingest if he becomes accustomed to eating everything sweetened. And the problem is the same if he gets used to eating sweeteners; in a few years' time, he will replace sweeteners with sugar.

Don't add any salt or sugar to the baby's food, but he can try food that contains them. It is all right for him to chew on bread (which contains salt) and biscuits (which contain sugar), or to eat our food.

Helpful (but not so important) hints

What follows are my personal opinions based on my experience as a parent and my personal preferences. But they are not based on scientific data, and each reader must decide if they agree with me or not.

What foods should you introduce first?

It doesn't matter. As we've explained earlier, there is no scientific basis to recommend one food over another. If you give your baby fruit first, followed by cereal, and then chicken, you will be abiding fully by the ESPGAN guidelines. But if you give chicken, then vegetables, then cereals, you will also be within the guidelines.

Let us suppose you begin with rice. Boil some rice, slightly overcook it if anything, and don't add salt. You can add a drop of olive oil (it will taste better and contain more calories). After you have breastfed her, offer your daughter one or two spoonfuls. It is best not to give her much more than that on the first day, even if she eats it gladly. If she refuses the first spoonful, don't insist, but try feeding it to her again every one or two days. If she wants, you can give her a little more every day. After a few days, try another food type, such as mashed banana. Later on, she can try boiled potato, chicken... This order is only used as an example, you can start in reverse, if you like. Of course, if one of these foods gives her diarrhoea or other symptoms, or if she rejects it vehemently, it is best to wait a few more weeks. If a more severe reaction is observed, like a rash, consult your doctor.

It is also not necessary to introduce a new food each week. For years we have been led to believe that variety is better (seven and a half types of cereals, thirteen with chocolate, fifteen with coffee…); this is merely a marketing strategy. Variety means some cereal, some legumes, some vegetables, some fruit – but it is not vital that baby eats lots of things from each food group. Apples don't have anything different than pears, and most adults manage quite well eating only two grains: rice and wheat, letting cattle eat the rest. If your child already eats chicken, you are not adding anything by introducing veal. Before one year, introducing many different foods only means buying more tickets for the allergy lottery.

The main reason for giving babies other foods at six months (and not later) is that some babies need extra iron. Therefore, it would seem logical that foods rich in iron be introduced first. On the one hand, there are meats with highly bio-available organic iron. On the other hand, you have vegetables, beans, and cereals that contain inorganic iron, which is harder to absorb unless it is paired with vitamin C. This is why many adults eat salad first (rich in vitamin C), then grains and legumes, and finally dessert. What we commonly do with babies in Spain is not such a great idea, giving them only grains at one meal, then vegetables at the next, and fruit at the next. When your baby eats several foods, it is a good idea to combine them, offering them at the same meal (not grinding them together), instead of making monochromatic menus ("time for cereal").

What if he doesn't want any food?

Do not worry; this is totally normal. Don't try to force him.

You may be told to feed solids before the breast so that the baby will be hungry enough to eat. This makes no sense because mother's milk nourishes much better than anything else. There is a reason we call solids "complementary foods"; solids do nothing more than to complement the breast. If your baby breastfeeds then rejects fruit, nothing happens; but if he eats fruit and then does not breastfeed, he is missing out. More fruit and less milk is a recipe for weight loss.

The same goes for formula. Remember that if you are not breastfeeding you must offer your baby 500 ml (17 oz) of milk each day until he is a year old. It is not good to hold back milk in order to get the baby to eat more solids.

Will he have all the nutrients he needs if I only feed him breastmilk?

Some babies after six months use up all the reserves of iron they had when they were born, and they need iron from other sources. This is one reason why we begin supplementing their diet. Others don't need to take iron until they are twelve months or older.

Many babies will only take breastmilk until eight or ten months, or older. They won't even try other food, and will spit out anything you put in their mouth. Will those babies develop an iron deficiency? Personally, I suppose they won't; if they refuse to eat, it is because they don't need to. However, there is no scientific research to back up this conviction. The opposite might also be the case: an iron deficiency produces a loss of appetite, and this explains why the baby isn't eating. On several occasions, I have seen babies of eight or ten months who only wanted breastmilk and who weren't putting on weight or were losing weight; they were found to be anaemic, and once they were given iron supplements, they began eating and putting on weight. It is good to introduce chicken and meat among the first solids you give your baby, because they are rich in iron (babies don't need large amounts). Also, don't give them fruit separately, they should eat it, like we do, after a meal; that way the vitamin C from the fruit helps them absorb the iron from the vegetables, legumes and cereals. If a baby refuses to eat and isn't putting on weight, it is a good idea to have him checked to make sure he doesn't have an iron deficiency, or some other illness. And what if he puts on weight without eating any solids? This means he has a good appetite and is taking a lot of breastmilk, in which case I assume he doesn't have an iron deficiency. However, if after several months he is still only taking breastmilk and the doctor or the parents are worried, there is no harm in having him tested.

You do not have to puree the food

Many mothers consult their doctor because their two- or three-year-old only wants pureed foods:

> *My child is five years old and he won't eat anything solid. He has always refused to chew. I have to spoon-feed him everything since he also refuses to feed himself.*

This is not really a severe problem, even if we did nothing, this child would end up eating normally. Or do you really think that at age fifteen he will still be eating pureed food? But it is a pain and it looks bad. Your baby will never get used to purees if he never tastes them. Soft foods like potato or cooked carrots, bananas, boiled rice, etc., can be mashed with a fork. Pears and apples can be grated. Firmer foods, like chicken, can be cut into miniature pieces with a knife, or you can ask your butcher to grind your chicken (be sure he adds nothing else) and then cook it in a small amount of oil and you'll have some beautiful mini chicken balls.

In this cruel age in which we live, many children have to go through three weanings instead of one. Every psychologist will tell you that weaning is a sensitive time and potentially traumatic. Yet many children wean first from the breast to the bottle before two months, then from the bottle to pureed foods around six months, and finally from pureed foods to normal foods around two or three years. And judging by the fighting and crying that goes on, each weaning is worse than the earlier one:

> *My son Juan, who is twenty months old, has always had trouble with changes; he has a hard time starting anything new. Switching from bottle to spoon was terrible, from sweet to salty the same, and so forth.*
>
> *At about a year we started introducing bigger pieces into his baby food, but he would only spit them out. So we let him keep eating smooth baby food, to this day. His molars just came through and even though he is well able to eat macaroni, crackers, potatoes, cereal, hot dogs, etc., he makes a game out of*

the whole thing, eating only a little in between meals. If we set a plate of cut-up food for him at mealtime, he just takes the food and throws it.

Why not wean a baby only once? From the breast to normal food, in a gradual process that starts at six months and can end several years down the road?

By the way, this mother has inadvertently come up with the solution: her son will eat pieces of food "as a game, between meals". That is, when he is not forced to eat. Once your child gets used to pureed food, trying to force him to eat other foods or making fun of him because he eats only pureed food will probably only make the situation worse. Do not force him to eat at all, whether it is pureed or regular food, and little by little he will start to try new things.

You do not have to prepare special foods

With a little planning, you can cook for your baby almost the same thing you would cook for the adults in your family. Cook without adding spices or salt, and add these things after taking out the baby's portion. For example:

Plain rice is an excellent gluten-free cereal for babies. Later on, you can add tomato sauce, which is a vegetable like any other (don't use ketchup, which isn't very suitable for a baby; homemade tomato sauce which contains only tomatoes and olive oil is fine).

There are a wide variety of cereals containing gluten: bread, noodles, semolina, alphabet soup, macaroni, spaghetti... To begin with he should be given them boiled with no sauce; later on you can cook them in a bouillon or season them with tomato sauce. Remember, a baby's stomach is small so giving him soup isn't a good idea: drain the alphabet soup, like miniature pasta.

Make sure you read the ingredients on the packet; cheap pasta is "100 percent durum wheat", but the more expensive one contains egg, and it is probably best to avoid giving this to babies with a family history of allergies. Similarly, ordinary bread only contains wheat, whereas some sliced breads or biscuits, depending on the make, also contain sugar, milk and eggs. For babies under one year simple foods are always better than ones with added ingredients.

If you look up "baby-led weaning" on the Internet, you will see dozens of babies eating the same as their parents from aged six months: spaghetti and rice with tomato sauce and broccoli and lentils. No more purees.

When mother works outside the home

I am worried because my three-month-old son won't accept a bottle. We've tried all sorts of nipples and different formulas. The doctor told me to stop breastfeeding so that he can get used to the bottle, but he's spent the last three days without eating and he still won't take it. I went back to breastfeeding, but I no longer have enough milk and he seems hungry even after feeding. What can I do to get him to take a bottle? I will be starting work soon and I have to wean him before then.

This mother was a victim of two frequent mistakes regarding breastfeeding and working.

The **first mistake** was to think that she had to wean her baby before going back to work. This is not necessary. In the worst case, she could do mixed feedings: breastfeeding before and after work, and formula feeding during the time she is away. All children (and all mothers) have a hard time when they must be separated because of work, and breastfeeding can be a wonderful way to make up for the separation and to reconnect. Many mothers find more satisfactory solutions rather than having to introduce formula: some take their baby to work, others job share, some have the baby brought to them for lunch, others express and store their milk. Better yet, if your baby is old enough for solids, have the child care provider feed solids to the baby when you are not there (this is the exception to the general rule of breastfeeding before solids).

When you go to work (or to walk the dog), your baby does

not know where you are or how long you will be gone. He will be very frightened and will cry as if you had left him forever. It will be several years before your baby will be able to be away from you without crying, and before he understands that "mummy will be right back". Any time you return, you hug him, breastfeed him, and the baby thinks "Whew, another false alarm!" But if you return to work and try to abruptly wean at the same time, then upon your return from work the baby will ask to be breastfed and you refuse; what then is baby to think? "Of course, she's abandoned me because she doesn't love me." It is a terrible time to wean.

The **second mistake** is to believe that if the baby is to be getting a bottle (or solids, for that matter) when you return to work, you must get him used to it first. If you manage to get him used to it, the only thing you will have accomplished is to borrow trouble: you could have achieved four months of exclusive breastfeeding, and now you've got only three. But what is relevant here is that, as we saw in the example above, on page 122, the baby many times refuses the bottle. Even when mothers express their milk and try to give that in the bottle, many babies refuse.

And the reason is that babies are no fools. If mother is not home and grandmother comes in with a bottle (or better yet with a cup to avoid nipple confusion), two things can happen. One, if baby is not very hungry, he may not drink a thing. He will make up for it when mother returns. Many babies spend most of their time away from mother sleeping, and then go on to nurse all night. This arrangement can be quite tolerable when mother and child share a bed, and many mothers find this a very good way to maintain a bond with their children in spite of long hours at work. The other possibility is that, if the baby is hungry (and especially if it is mother's milk in the bottle), he may take it, and that's it. Inside he may be thinking: "Well, she's not here, so this will have to do."

But if mother is home and the baby can see and smell the breast, how is he going to accept a cup or bottle? He must think: "My mother must be crazy, she's got the breast right there and she wants to give me this contraption?" No wonder he insists, "It's the breast or nothing!"

Myths surrounding solid foods

Myth – baby food is more nutritious than milk alone.

This is such a common misconception that, even though we've already alluded to it, it seems necessary to restate. Many mothers are told that "their milk is no longer nourishing" or that "your milk is water". Such phrases can seem like an insult similar to calling someone "empty headed" or "heartless". The bad thing is that there are people who believe it. Let's get real, please! There are no women who have water instead of milk, just as there are no flying elephants.

Let's look at a real situation:

> My daughter is six months old. During this time she has been and continues to be breastfed. However I started solids (fruits and cereal) at four months as my doctor suggested.
>
> Up until her fourth month my baby had been growing beautifully, weighing 6.3 kg (13 lbs 14 oz) and was 63 cm long (24.5 in), but at her last doctor's visit she only weighed 6.980 kg (15 lbs 6 oz) and was 66 cm long (26 in). The doctor has told me to wean her from the breast and put her on the following schedule: 9:00 am cereal, 1:00 pm vegetables, 5:30 pm fruit, and 9:30 pm cereal.

What is strange about this case? Not the weight, that is normal at four months and is still normal at six. The amount gained in this period is also normal. What is strange (or should be) is the diagnosis by the doctor and stranger still is the treatment suggested.

If the doctor was right and if the weight gain were insufficient, and if the cause were poor nutrition, then the logical reasoning should go like this: what was she eating when she was gaining well? Exclusive breastfeeding. What was she eating when she stopped gaining well? Mother's milk and solids. Conclusion: remove the solids, quick. Instead, what is chosen is to run full steam ahead, wean from the breast and don't even trade it in for the bottle. This baby is six months old, and only eating four times a day, once only fruit and once only vegetables. Although we know now that babies do not need as many calories as once was thought, this diet doesn't even cover the minimum. Luckily, this mother switched doctors and the second doctor gave her a diet that, although not ideal to recover full breastfeeding, at least allowed for the survival of this child (a bottle of formula instead of vegetables, and nursing after every meal).

Being a staunch defender of breastfeeding (can you tell?), I am tempted to say that this child is gaining slowly because of the early introduction of solids. But this would not be true. She is gaining slowly, not due to what she eats or not, but because of her age. Even if she had been exclusively breastfed the entire time, she would have gained the same. Even if the parents had fed her pork and beans and chocolate cake for dessert she would have gained the same (or maybe less because the food might not have agreed with her).

All children gain more during the first three months, while they are only breastfeeding (or bottle-feeding), than they do during the second three months. From six to nine months, with a little bit of solids, they gain even less, and from nine months to one year, with a lot more solid food, they almost don't gain at all. All doctors have seen this hundreds and thousands of times. However, many still seem convinced that solids fatten babies up better than milk. I wonder where this belief came from.

As we have said before, baby food containing meat and vegetables often has fewer calories than milk, not to mention just vegetables or fruit alone. Of course, some solids, such as cereals do have more calories. But what about proteins and the quality of those proteins? What about vitamins, minerals, essential fatty acids, and other nutrients? Would you say that flour is more nutritious than milk?

Our diet must satisfy a whole range of needs. The only food capable of satisfying all the needs of the human body, all by itself, at least during one part of our life is human milk. A newborn is perfectly well nourished during six or more months with only human milk. But nobody would be well nourished in infancy or in any other stage of life by eating only meat, only bread, or only oranges. Not to say that meat, bread and oranges are not nutritious, it is just that they need to be complemented by other foods. Complemented, not substituted.

Of course, we cannot only drink human milk for our entire life and at a certain point human milk must be complemented with other foods. But let us not be misled, the main reason we do not drink human milk our entire life is that no one would give it to us. Although perhaps not perfect, mother's milk is the closest thing to the perfect food, at any age, more than any other known food. A castaway on a deserted island could survive longer if he only had human milk than if he only had bread, or only apples, or only chickpeas, or only meat.

If some ignorant fool says to you, "Wean him from the breast, your milk no longer has enough protein," you can answer them: "Well then, I'll also have to take away fruits and vegetables since they have even less protein." And if someone says your milk is water you can respond: "Of course, that's why I give it to him, it is pure water, not like tap water with so much chlorine." On second thoughts, perhaps you'd better not say anything; some fools don't have much of a sense of humour.

Myth – with a good solid food feeding before bed, he'll sleep all night.

Well, no. Many children continue to wake every night even at two or three years old, even if they had potatoes and eggs or beans with sausage for dinner.

It has been demonstrated, that children do not sleep more when they have more solids.[33] During their first years children wake at night, not only because they need to eat, but also because they need us. Luckily, breastfeeding allows us to satisfy both these needs at the same time, and the child goes back to sleep quickly, so much so that some parents call the breast "anaesthesia".

Myth – after six months babies should drink "follow-up milk."

Follow-on milk (also known as follow-up milks in some countries) is a commercial invention, without practical use. In the United States, the American Academy of Pediatrics (AAP) recommends feeding non-breastfed infants the same milk for the entire first year of a baby's life. The World Health Organization (WHO) also believes that follow-on milks are unnecessary.

Why were these milks invented then? There is a very simple explanation. The law in many countries (Spain included) bans the advertising of formula for babies younger than six months. But the majority of countries, unfortunately, do not prohibit the advertising of follow-on milks (advertised for babies from six months on). For the formula manufacturers it is ideal to have two milks by the same name that are only differentiated by a little number. Is there anyone so naïve as to believe that publicity for "Badmilk 2" will not increase the sales of "Badmilk 1"?

The main advantage of follow-on milks, according to the ESPGAN, is that they are cheaper. Since formula designed to meet the needs of young babies can be expensive, low-income mothers might be tempted to introduce regular milk before one year, which would not be best. Having, instead, formula for an older baby, which is cheaper, because it is not adapted to the needs of a younger baby, could be of help for some families.

Not as adapted? Sure. Cow's milk has excess proteins, more than three times those in human milk. This is one of its greatest dangers: a baby cannot metabolize such a large amount of protein and could become severely ill. Making formula involves several steps, one of which is to remove the majority of the proteins. It is not easy to remove proteins from milk. If you don't have to remove as much protein, it becomes easier to make, and therefore less expensive. The ESPGAN seems to think that the difference in price would be significant, but at least in Spain, the difference to the consumer is negligible.

It is not that follow-up milks are better for older babies. They are actually worse than start-up milks since they are less modified. Older babies, however, are better able to metabolize and tolerate them. Naturally, the infant food industry tries to use the higher protein content in their publicity, so they advertise their follow-up milks as: "Enriched with proteins to meet the growing needs of your baby."

What stupidity! The need for protein actually diminishes as the child grows,[10] going from 2 g (0.07 oz) per 1 kg of weight per day at birth to 0.89 g (0.03 oz) between six and nine months, and 0.82 g (0.02 oz) between nine and twelve months. A child weighing 8 kg (17 lbs 10 oz) needs 7.12 g (0.25 oz) of protein a day. He can obtain that through 790 ml (27 oz) of human milk per day (a totally reasonable intake) or with 550 ml (19 oz) of artificial start-up formula (which always has a little more protein than human milk to try to compensate for its inferior quality). This same baby, drinking 500 ml (17 oz) of follow-up milk would receive 11 g (0.4 oz) of protein, much more than his body needs, without taking into account the protein in the cereals or chicken that he might eat.

Do not be taken in by publicity. The excess proteins in follow-up milks are not any good for your child; they are simply industrial waste.

Children who breastfeed should keep breastfeeding. The AAP recommends that babies get human milk for at least the first year and thereafter "as long as is mutually desired." The WHO and UNICEF recommend breastfeeding for "two years or beyond".[34]

Naturally, if for whatever reason you want to wean your child before a year, you will have to give him some other milk, be it start-up or follow-up formula. The decision is yours. Do not allow others to choose for you. No bottle-feeding mother has ever been told: "This milk no longer nourishes, starting now you are to give him only human milk, or prepare his cereal using human milk." It is understood that when a mother decides to bottle-feed, she will do so for years. A breastfeeding mother deserves the same respect.

Myth – if he doesn't eat meat he won't get enough protein.

We just finished explaining this: even if the baby only drank milk, he would still have enough protein. Cereals and legumes add even more proteins. In spite of this, some mothers become intimidated by strange arguments:

> *I am a mostly vegetarian mother although I occasionally eat some fish. I would like to raise my daughter the same way. Those who disagree with me argue that meat is necessary to build muscle tissue, etc.*

The other day, at the zoo, I saw a rhinoceros. I was told it never eats any meat. He seemed to have a lot of strong muscle tissue. Of course, I did not get too near; perhaps once you got close enough to touch him, you'd find out he's all flabby.

Chapter 9
What the healthcare provider can do

"My child won't eat" is one of the most frequent complaints doctors hear.[35] Health professionals are in a wonderful position to prevent infant feeding problems or to help parents avert them in their initial stages, before they become a source of conflict and anguish for the family.

However, sometimes our advice, even our passing comments, can contribute to or aggravate the problem. Two aspects of our performance are especially susceptible: weight checks and the introduction of solids.

Weight checks

I have a three-month-old baby girl. She weighed 3 kg (6 lbs 10 oz) at birth. From the first day I breastfed her and she's been gaining very well until about a month ago. At that time, she only gained 40 g (1.4 oz) in two weeks.

The doctor said that mother's milk was no longer enough and that I should supplement with 60 ml (2 oz) of formula after breastfeeding five minutes on each side. This is where the problems started, since my daughter would not take the bottle. I was trying not to force her, leaving her alone when she rejected the bottle, and insisting at the next feeding. She never wanted the bottle. We tried different brands of formula, different teats, and we even sweetened the milk. Nothing worked. The next week, my daughter had gained 260 g (9 oz) so the doctor agreed to let me just breastfeed since she'd gone back to normal. But last week she only gained 20 g (less than an ounce) and so he told me to breastfeed at one feeding and bottle-feed for the next.

But the baby still refuses. I only manage to get her upset and she won't stop crying. I've also tried the bottle for every feeding so that she realizes there is no more breastfeeding and finally she might take it, but it has been in vain. She would rather go without food; after a while she just cries herself to sleep.

I am desperate; I don't know what to do. I also tried putting my own milk in the bottle and that did work. After that, I tried to mix my milk with the formula, but she rejected that. To get her to eat, when she's nursing, I try to drizzle some formula in the corner of her mouth. But I only manage to have her drink lots of air and little milk.

In one short month, happy and relaxed mothering has become a nightmare. The diagnostic process was wrong. The weight gain was evaluated in too short a time span and it was compared with inappropriate reference numbers. And the treatment has been unnecessary and incorrect. If a baby is fully breastfeeding, the answer would not be to add bottles, but to increase breastfeeding.

The intrinsic variability of growth, the errors in measuring, and the variations caused by the time since the last feeding, as well as voiding and elimination make the weekly weight check totally useless. This is evident in the example above, where this baby, without changing her diet (since she did not take the bottle) can gain 20 g (less than an ounce) or 260 g (9 oz). As Fomon[2] states: "Weight increases at intervals shorter than one month must be interpreted with caution" during the first six months. In the second six months, weight gain is assessed in two-month intervals.

A standard weight chart and a growth velocity chart are not the same thing. Weight charts monitor the weight at a given time, but not the increase in weight over a span of time. When growth seems either abnormally fast or slow, you should consult a baby growth chart. As well as their child-growth standards, the WHO has also brought out weight velocity tables in periods of one, two, three, four and six months. These are based on the growth of normal children who receive normal nourishment (that is breastmilk). For the first two months, the WHO growth charts are divided into periods of one or two weeks, differentiated according to weight at birth. All of these are available at www.who.int/childgrowth/standards/en.

In four weeks, between age two and three months, this baby has gained a total of 320 g (11.2 oz), which is above the 5th percentile in Nelson's charts (260 g or 9 oz in 28 days), and above the –2 deviation on the WHO charts (280 g or 9.9 oz in one month). Therefore, this weight gain is totally normal. Keep in mind that the –2 deviation in the growth chart is not the same as the difference in actual weight in the –2 deviation; in this case, the weight that corresponds to the –2 deviation is 3.810 kg (8 lbs 6 oz) at two months of age and 4.380 kg (9 lbs 10 oz) at three months with an increase of 570 g (1 lb 4 oz). The use of standard weight charts (that show attained weight) instead of growth velocity charts (that show weight increases) produces huge mistakes when making calculations.

Also, as Fomon adds, in populations where malnutrition is low, the majority of infants whose weight increase over a certain period falls below the 5th percentile are normal (obviously, as 5 percent of babies will gain weight under the 5th percentile).

This mother and baby would have been better off had the weight been measured at longer intervals, and the excessive therapeutic enthusiasm given way to prudent observation. Besides, this baby's staunch refusal of the bottle confirms she was not hungry (although the opposite is not always true; many babies younger than two or three months will take a bottle even when they are not hungry). In a vain attempt at trying to wean the child from the breast in order to get her to take the bottle, she is doing neither, eating even less than before the foolish advice was given.

In the case of Herminia's son we see again the importance of using the appropriate reference:

My son is now ten months old. He was born at 3.950 kg (8 lbs 11 oz). He has always been breastfed and was growing fine until about two months ago, when he's fallen below the mean.

Two different doctors have advised me to supplement with formula since my milk no longer nourishes him, but my baby refuses. He doesn't want to even smell it and I fear he will never accept it and that not only will he not gain, but may also start losing weight. I feel terrible about this since I wanted to continue breastfeeding for at least a year and a half.

At six months my baby weighed 8.170 kg (18 lbs), but at nine months he was only 8.950 kg (19 lbs 11 oz) and at ten months 9.260 kg (20 lbs 6 oz). He is 76 cm (29.5 in) long.

Herminia's son gained 410 g (14.5 oz) between eight and ten months. We consulted the weight velocity table for two months' increments. Between eight and ten months, the average weight gain is 544 g (19 oz), and the 3rd percentile is 60 g for the two months together! Not only is his weight gain within the norm, if anything it is higher, above the 25th percentile (360 g or 12.5 oz). This child's absolute refusal to feed from a bottle confirms that his weight gain isn't due to not having enough milk.

It is quite normal for weight gain in any given month to be in the 10th or the 3rd percentile, or even lower. All the percentiles, from the first to the hundredth, are normal, because the charts and standards are elaborated exclusively with data from healthy children. But that month where weight gain is only in the 3rd percentile is as a rule an exception, an inconsistency that could be caused by a virus, an attack of diarrhoea, a separation from the mother, or an extreme variation in a process that is by nature erratic. In these cases, the baby will normally gain more weight the following month. That is why there are charts for periods of differing lengths of time, and it is essential to use the most appropriate one. Let us look at an example from the WHO charts:

Girls, growth in periods of one month, 3rd percentile:
3–4 months: 214 g [7.5 oz]
4–5 months: 130 g [4.6 oz]
5–6 months: 52 g [1.8 oz]
6–7 months: −4 g [−0.1 oz]

Does this mean a healthy girl can only gain 214 + 130 + 52 – 4 = 392 g between the ages of three and seven months? No, because a healthy child can gain "the minimum" in any given month, but not for several months in a row.

Now let us look at another chart:

Girls, growth in periods of two months, 3rd percentile:
3–5 months: 556 g [16.6 oz]
5–7 months: 267 g [9.4 oz]

The total is 823 grams, more than double the total for four periods of one month. But that still isn't enough:

Girls, growth in periods of four months, 3rd percentile:
3–7 months: 1071 g [7.5 oz]

It is therefore essential to evaluate the whole – the increase over the whole period – and not simply to look at the monthly growth. It is also important to take height into account; the normal weight for a short child may be too little for a taller child.

Starting solids

My doctor has advised me to start feeding my baby gluten-free cereal twice a day. The problem is that my son (four-and-a-half months) doesn't want anything to do with it, and the doctor has told me I must make him. This is very frustrating and my heart breaks to see how hard it is for the baby. Since birth he has never been one to eat a lot; many times being satisfied with only a couple of minutes at the breast and he has never accepted a bottle.

Even though the most updated recommendations are to start solids after six months and not at four,[20] here it is not the timing of the introduction of foods that has initiated conflict, but the advice to force the child to eat. Remember that foods should be introduced in small amounts and increased slowly, following the baby's cues.

Teresa's story is even more dramatic:

At six-and-a-half months we started fruit and things were worse than with cereal. He refused them from the start; he would turn his head and clamp his mouth closed at the sight of the spoon. If by chance I could manage to get anything in his mouth, he spat it out. So I had to keep on breastfeeding.

When I went in for his seven-month checkup, the doctor fussed at me and told me I had to be firm with my son and, if he refused to eat his cereal or fruit, that I should not offer the breast even if he cried and was hungry. I was supposed to only offer water until the next meal. Although the baby was growing fine, the doctor said I should have done more to get him to eat. He explained that now my baby had come into a much more active stage where he would need more energy and carbohydrates from cereals as well as the vitamins and minerals that come from fruits.

Teresa's son at seven months is 72.5 cm long (28.5 in) and weighs 9 kg (19 lbs 13 oz). According to the WHO charts, his height is well above the 85th percentile, his weight is closer to the 85th than to the 50th percentile, and his ratio weight/height is exactly average. In light of these numbers, although Teresa does not tell us his weight gain in the past few months, it is highly unlikely that there were any problems. In fact, the child's refusing to eat is more than enough proof that he was not hungry. Not to mention the illogical advice to give water instead of milk because of higher energy requirements: water does not add any calories. Complementary feeding is not meant to substitute for breastfeeding, only to complement it. Besides, as we have said before, the energy needs per 1 kg (2.2 lbs) of weight do not increase, but decrease throughout the baby's first year.

Watch your language

Words, once uttered, cannot be taken back and the stories of many mothers throughout this book show us the distress that even a casual comment may generate.

Health care professionals must ban from their language expressions such as "barely on the chart" or "slow to gain" and "not gaining well". Either the child meets the criteria for failure to thrive[2] (weight gain below the −2 deviation for at least two months if younger than six months or for three months if older than three months; and the height/weight ratio below the 5th percentile), or he doesn't. Of course, in some borderline cases it is smart to watch the weight carefully, and perhaps recommend more frequent feedings; but this can be done without labelling the child and worrying the parents.

Doctors can also make recommendations in a more casual way. Compare the following phrases:

- "Starting at x months, give the baby chicken."
- "Starting at x months, you can start offering chicken."
- "In the evening, give 180 ml (6 oz) of pureed vegetables."
- "When it is convenient for you, offer some vegetables. Increase the amount if the baby takes them happily."

Strict recommendations on amounts, schedules, the order of the introduction of foods, and other details are not based on science,[2,18] but can conflict with the baby's needs, the mother's opinion, and her family's customs as well as the advice from other professionals.

Finally, it is at least somewhat disturbing that a mother can leave a health care provider's office with the feeling that he "fussed at" her.

Take the scale off the pedestal

Well-baby exams often follow a kind of protocol. The mother explains how the child is doing while she undresses him. Then the paediatrician does his exam. Finally he weighs and measures the child and then and only then does the mother ask: "So, how's he doing, doctor?"

It would seem that the child's weight is the only important measure of the child's health.

What really matters is what the mother says. She is the one who sees the child every day. Next in importance is the exam, which allows the doctor to determine the baby's physical health and development. And of least importance is the weight, which rarely gives us information that we did not already suspect: if a child is really malnourished or obese, you can see it. The main usefulness in weighing the child is to simply have a reference number, should the child become ill later on, to be able to see exactly how much weight has been lost.

Is there anything health care providers can do to alter the scale's place at the centre of the surgery visit? Perhaps, instead of waiting to weigh the child before saying he's "okay", we could start by restating what we hear the mother say:

"So, according to what you're saying, your daughter is healthy and developing normally."

Then, during the exam, we could go on explaining: "She tracks very well with her eyes. Her chest sounds normal."

And then, finally: "Your child is wonderfully healthy and strong. Now, just to satisfy our curiosity, let's see how much she weighs."

Part IV
Frequently asked questions

What if he really *doesn't eat?*

Of course there are children who do not eat, that is, who eat less than what their body needs. The difference between a child who does not eat from one who "does not eat" is that the first loses weight while the second does not.

The reasons behind a child really not eating are varied. Some are similar to those that make adults stop eating: getting sick with a cold or flu, diarrhoea, sore throat, not to mention more serious illnesses.

If the child is not eating because he has tuberculosis, he will not get better by being stuffed with food. He will get better when he receives the appropriate treatment for his illness, and once he is well, he will start to eat on his own. So the same general rule still applies: Never force your child to eat. If he is healthy, he has eaten what he needs. If he is sick, offer his favourite foods frequently, but without forcing him to eat or he'll end up throwing up. If he loses weight, take him to the doctor:

> *I exclusively breastfed Cristina (now-seven-and-a-half months) for six months and then started offering solids, without making her eat. But now she won't eat. The doctor tells me that she has stopped growing and that I must wean her so that she will eat. She has been nursing every hour-and-a-half for the past two months.*

141

Cristina failed to gain weight from five to eight months. The mother, Marisa, went to several doctors who all agreed that the problem was that the chld was "spoiled" by breastfeeding so frequently. Weaning was the only option to get her to eat. Between eight and nine months this baby not only failed to gain, but she lost weight so the mother took her to the emergency department at a good hospital. The diagnosis was cystic fibrosis, a severe inherited disease. This is an extreme example, but unfortunately it is not all that rare. If the breastfed baby fails to gain, no one worries, no one does any testing, no one bothers to figure out what might be wrong. The mother is simply told to wean. Then, when the baby also fails to gain on the bottle, the doctors really start to worry and often discover that the baby is actually sick. It is sad, but some mothers find themselves having to lie and hide the fact that they are still breastfeeding in order to obtain the necessary medical attention for their child.

Curiously enough, the only food that Cristina would eat, other than mother's milk (thankfully this mother did not follow the foolish advice to wean!), was chicken. I believe that this just goes to show that children really do know what they need; cystic fibrosis patients lose proteins, and Cristina was looking for foods rich in protein.

Other children stop eating for psychological reasons. I once saw a little girl, just over one year, who refused to eat and lost weight quickly when her mother returned to work. The child had two grandmothers, one who visited often and played with the baby. However, for a variety of reasons, the mother had chosen the other grandmother as the babysitter, a woman who the baby barely knew. The baby had found herself suddenly "abandoned" by her mother and in the hands of a complete stranger. (I know that the mother did not abandon her, but the baby didn't know it, could not know it. During the first few years, when mothers are separated from their babies even for just a few hours, children behave as if mother were gone forever.)

Do I have to wean in order to get my baby to eat?

My daughter was born seven-and-a-half months ago. Since then she has never left the breast. Every feeding I prepare and offer her baby food, yet she turns her head and won't open her mouth for anything. What can I do? Should I wean her entirely as some suggest in order for her to eat?

Just like Marisa (see pages 141–2), many mothers are told that weaning will make their baby start eating food. As if bottle-fed babies ate so well!

I am a desperate mother. My ten-month-old daughter only wants to drink from her bottle and of course, she hates vegetables.

As we have explained (see the section "When mother works outside the home" on page 122), abrupt weaning can easily produce a rejection of solids. On occasion, I have seen a baby lose 500 g (1 lb 1 oz) in one week when mother attempts abrupt weaning. Upon returning the baby to breastfeeding (what both mother and child were hoping for), he immediately recovers his interest in life and starts to take not only the breast, but sometimes also the bottle. Having recovered the lost weight, the baby may easily return to exclusive breastfeeding. In other situations, when no one intervenes to help the mother and baby, the baby ends up giving up and taking the bottle, since the survival instinct is stronger than anything. After baby accepts the bottle he will recover the lost weight, but often remains "slow to gain".

Do you think I'm making this up? Read what happened to Laura:

My eleven-month-old daughter weighs 7.230 kg (15 lbs 15 oz) and is 71 cm (27.9 in). The problem is she does not want to eat. I breastfed her for eight months. At four months old I introduced fruit and at five months cereal; after that we did vegetables with meat and fish. Her weight was fine until her six-month checkup. Since then she has eaten very little and lately she practically doesn't eat at all.

While we were still nursing, she seemed interested in food, but now mealtimes have become agony.

According to the Spanish and American charts that were in use when she was small, Laura's weight was below the 3rd percentile (which is not necessarily abnormal, as I already mentioned). Someone must have thought she would gain more weight on formula. Evidently, she didn't. According to the WHO charts, Laura's weight is normal, a quarter of a kilo (9 oz) above the 3rd percentile. However, the problem isn't which of the charts we consult: the old ones can be used with caution and common sense, while those of the WHO can be used in a rigid or unthinking way.

What if she has anorexia?

Anorexia nervosa is a severe mental illness. It does not occur in small children, but in adolescents (although we are starting to see it in younger and younger patients). In any case, you don't cure it by making the patient eat, because this would be counterproductive. So our rule still stands: do not force a child to eat and if there is weight loss look for illness (which may also be mental). Adolescents with anorexia lose weight. They lose a lot of weight. Therefore, if your child has not lost weight, no matter her age, she does not have anorexia nervosa.

Could she have infantile anorexia?

I agree with all you write, but in the case of my daughter it does not apply; she really does not eat.

From the start she refused the breast. I had to express my milk and bottle-feed her. But then my milk dried up and we started formula feeding (and the suffering). She would drink half the bottle and then just cry. They did all sorts of lab tests and all came out fine although she seemed to have a little reflux so they gave her medication (cisapride) and a special reflux milk. The only way she would eat was while she was asleep.

She is now thirteen months old and weighs 7 kg (15 lbs 6 oz) and things are awful. She barely drinks any milk. She'll only take four or five bites of solids.

The doctor is talking about admitting her to the hospital and using a feeding tube, so that she'll gain weight, and then to start psychological counselling.

The doctors have ruled out any organic cause.

Let us make clear that the term "anorexia" means, "lacking in appetite" or "not eating". This is a symptom that can accompany almost any illness. A child with a sore throat, or an adult with diarrhoea, will probably also have anorexia. However, anorexia nervosa is a specific disease. It's the same as the difference between "a fever", a common symptom in hundreds of different illnesses, or "typhoid fever", a specific and concrete disease. There is no illness called "infantile anorexia"; it's simply a fancy way of saying that "the child won't eat".

Let's say you take your child to the doctor saying that you notice he's been very hot; the doctor, after checking him over, might say, "He has an ear infection." He has given you a diagnosis, information that you lacked. But if all he says is, "He has a fever", you might reply: "Well, I already knew that, but I still don't know the cause." In the same way, if you say, "My child won't eat" and someone tells you, "He has infantile anorexia", they have not diagnosed a thing. They have simply repeated, using a mix of Greek and Latin, what you just said.

Going back to the thirteen-month-old baby girl, Maite, described on page 144: it is true that this baby's weight is under the last line of the chart, but not too far below. What makes sense is for the doctor to do tests to make sure she is not sick. But if everything comes back normal, we have proven that this baby is healthy, totally healthy. Therefore we have one of the 15,000 (3 percent of the total) healthy babies in Spain, who at one year old are under the 3rd percentile. (In the United States, there are 200,000 babies below the 5th percentile.)

The idea of feeding her using a tube is ridiculous. Unfortunately this is not the first time I have heard this. I am not shy about saying that this is a form of abuse and that you'd really have to "start psychological counselling" if you were to subject the child to this cruelty. Just as it is not ethical to take someone's appendix out unless he is sick, it is not right to admit a child to the hospital and tube-feed her when she is healthy. And Maite is healthy; this has been proven by all the tests that have been normal.

If Maite were to continue to lose weight for unknown reasons, even after having all the normal results from the tests; if she went down to 6 kg (13 lbs 4 oz) and then to 5 and 4 kg (11 or 9 lbs), if she were to lose her interest in life and start to look like a snuffed-out candle, then you could logically say: "We didn't find anything wrong, but she's obviously sick. Let's use a feeding tube or, in a desperate attempt to keep this child alive, intravenous therapy. All this while we keep trying to find out what's really wrong in the hope that we can save her or that some miracle happens and she gets better on her own." However, Maite has been gaining weight consistently, albeit slowly, since birth, her motor development is normal and, when not tortured into eating, she is a happy child.

By the way, cisapride is almost never used anymore and has been taken off the market in the United States because of its serious side effects. Regarding reflux milks, they have been found not to be helpful even when there is a genuine reflux diagnosis.[36]

What would have happened if Maite, instead of being born now, in the age of socialized medicine and free unlimited paediatrician's visits in Spain, had been born in the last century? Someone might have noticed she was skinny and perhaps her mother might have given her one of the many "constitutional tonics" that were advertised at the time. But no one would have done tests, the parents would not have been frightened, and no one would have threatened to tube-feed her. If they had checked with Dr. Ulecia y Cardona, a reputed specialist in the treatment of malnourished children (whom you will meet in the Appendix), he would have been unconcerned.[43] In his book we see pictures of the children he treated with success: T.A., six-and-a-half months, weighing 4.020 kg (8 lbs 13 oz) and reaching 5.530 kg (12 lbs

3 oz) by thirteen months; M.C., sixteen months and weighing 5.800 kg (12 lbs 13 oz) and at two years doing "very well" because he reached 7.700 kg (16 lbs 15 oz). These were weight problems, and all were treated without feeding tubes, only with appropriate food.

Won't his stomach shrink?

No. Sorry, I know that in a book like this you probably expect a longer answer. But words fail me. Simply: no.

What if he's just doing it to get attention?

"Getting attention" is an unfortunate expression. Different people understand it in different, even opposite ways, and for an expression there is no bigger misfortune.

In common vernacular "to get attention" means to do things to get people to notice you. You may dye your hair green, or walk around with a tiger on a leash. In this sense, getting attention is considered totally negative, similar to "looking like a fool" or "acting up". No one pays much attention to those who merely seek to "get attention".

To psychologists who study child behaviour, "getting attention" has at least two distinct meanings, and neither is negative. It never means that the child is just "making a fool of himself", "acting up", or that you should ignore him.

The first meaning of this phrase refers to a spontaneous (instinctive) behaviour common to other mammal species: when a youngster becomes separated from his mother to play or explore, he frequently returns to let her know where he is and what he's up to. At the same time, the mother frequently looks for her offspring and calls out to him by making sounds, when she is about to move off, or if he wanders too far. Among non-human mammals, this takes place through barking, growling, or bleating but among humans it takes on more complex nuances: "Mummy, look at the castle I made!", "Judy, stay on the pavement!", "Look, Mummy, I'm a pirate!", "Come on, Pablo, time to go!"

It is easy to see that getting mother's attention has contributed for millions of years to the survival of our species. Youngsters who did not constantly get the attention of the adults got lost or were eaten and thus were eliminated by natural selection. Getting our attention in this way is an instinct in our children; they can't help it, and if we yell at them to leave us alone because we want to read the paper, we only manage to make them feel insecure and therefore want to get our attention even more.

The second meaning psychologists give to the expression "getting attention" refers to the more or less irregular behaviour that takes place when a person needs attention and does not know how to obtain it in the usual ways. So it is said that a child who bangs his head, throws up, kicks, or soils his pants may be trying to get attention. Adults also do things to get attention: they get hysterical, threaten or attempt suicide, shout, or fight. No one reaches these extremes unless easier methods to get attention (like talking or crying) have failed.

When a psychologist says, "This child hits or bites to get attention", what he means is: "This child needs much more attention than he is getting and has resorted to hitting or biting because no one pays attention unless he behaves in this way; you must give him a lot of attention to solve the problem." Unfortunately, many parents, and even some specialists, understand this expression as it is used commonly, like "this child is being foolish" or "he's acting up", and thus they think that they must ignore the behaviour to make it stop.

The majority of children who refuse to eat do it simply because they do not need more food. The only attention they intend to get is to let us know that "Hey, I'm finished eating!" It is possible that some child looks to get attention at mealtime regarding other things and this would show us that he needs more attention: someone to play with him, read him stories, respect his small achievements, and not to deny him physical contact and companionship. Of course, he also needs not to be forced to eat.

Does he need water, juice, or tea?

I was told in the hospital that I should give my baby water, especially in the summer. The thing is the baby (one year old) does not want to drink water. She won't drink water from a bottle; she takes a few sips from the cup and then just plays with it. We have tried to make her drink and she just slaps the bottle away. I have tried juices both homemade and store-bought but she doesn't like them. How can I make drinking water more attractive to her?

I'm sorry; there is no way to make a child drink water. If she needed water, she would drink it; if she does not drink it, it is because she does not need it. Period.

Children who are exclusively breastfed on demand do not need water, unless they have a high fever or diarrhoea (in this case you must breastfeed frequently and then perhaps offer some water after nursing). Studies have been done with Bedouins in the desert. These babies do not need water.

Bottle-fed babies who are fed on demand with appropriately prepared formula do not need extra water either. It's amazing how many people, health professionals included, still believe they do. If experts say, "one scoop of powder for every 30 ml (1 oz) of water", then it's for a reason. If formula-fed babies needed more water, the experts could just as easily say, "one scoop for every 40 ml (1.3 oz) of water".

After starting solids, if what the child is eating is mostly fruit and vegetables, he probably needs even less water than before. When children start eating more food that is saltier or dryer (chicken, bread, crackers), they will start to get thirsty.

Just in case, when you start solids, you can start to offer water in a cup (breastfed babies will prefer the cup to a bottle; and bottle-fed infants might as well start learning). But if your child doesn't drink the water, don't insist. He knows what he needs to drink, don't doubt his judgment.

It is very important that you only offer water to drink. Not juice, not tea, not sugar water; only water. Habitual juice and soft drink consumption instead of water is one of the causes of childhood and youth obesity that is so prevalent these days.

Fruit is very healthy, but juice is not as good for children. Not that store-bought juice contains anything evil; it doesn't. Even if you make it at home, it is best to limit juice consumption. The problem is that one cup of juice takes at least two oranges. Few people eat two oranges in one sitting. But juice is so easy to drink, first one glass, and then another until some children consume more than one litre (33.8 oz) of juice in one day. Small stomachs get full of juice and then they can't eat anything else. Older children have the opposite problem in that their stomach is larger, and they can fit all they need to eat plus the juice, which produces obesity. At any age, the excess of natural sugar in fruit may produce chronic diarrhoea. This is why the American Academy of Pediatrics (AAP)[37] recommends waiting on juice until after six months. Between one year and six years, the maximum intake (maximum, since they don't need any) would be between 110 and 170 ml per day (4 and 6 oz). And between six and eighteen years, twice that amount. In other words, for a party, juice is better than soft drinks of course; but for daily consumption, offer only water.

Regarding instant teas for babies (which are common in many countries), it is a shame they are not taken off the market. They are made up of 95 percent sugar, usually glucose (dextrose) and in some cases sucrose (table sugar). If you gave your baby the amount of tea recommended on the label, by the time he was one year old, he would have ingested more than 7 kg (15 lbs) of pure sugar. If babies needed these infusions (which they do not), it would be better to make them at home, without sugar, and if they needed sugar (which they do not), you could buy it at any store for 40 times less.

Why do they throw up so much?

I am a desperate twenty-four-year old mother. My daughter is eleven months old and she's never been a good eater. To top this off, she frequently throws up. When she was tiny, the doctor blamed it on reflux and switched her from human milk to anti-reflux formula. But we still have problems. Out of four meals, she throws up two. I was told that I was feeding her too much, but by the time she got to the fifth bite she'd throw up. Everything gags her. She refuses anything hard, like a cracker, and as soon as she gets anything chunky in her mouth, she throws up. I've tried making all her food smooth and she still throws up; she even throws up the milk she drinks. I'm now trying commercial baby food and she still throws up with those. She's had all sorts of tests done and I've been told that everything checks out as normal. But it seems impossible to me that she's never hungry and that she continues to gain even if she eats nothing all day.

It has been a nightmare; I don't get to enjoy my baby like other mothers because I am so worried. How long is this going to last?

It is easy to understand Manuela's concern. She doesn't say how much her daughter weighs, but it must be normal since she's "been told that everything checks out as normal". In other words, even though Manuela thinks her daughter has eaten very little, it is clear she has eaten too much. Even after throwing up, she's taken in enough to grow and develop normally without getting sick.

All babies spit up. Some only a little, and others a lot. Doctors call this gastroesophageal reflux (GER), in other words, the food that was in the stomach is coming back up. In the great majority of cases (unless the baby is losing weight, throwing up blood, or something else like that), it is something totally normal. Babies have the opening to their stomach open, and food will come out. Around one year it starts to close and they stop spitting up.

Unless, of course, they are forced to eat. As we have explained, when you try to feed a baby more than he needs, he throws up. He can't help it.

What if we are vegetarians?

Children as well as adults can live perfectly well with an ovo-lacto vegetarian diet.[33]

More limited vegetarian diets (without eggs or milk) can be adequate for a child, as long as he is breastfed for two or three years and as long as appropriate foods are combined in his diet. It is beyond the scope of this book to go into more detail. It would not be very smart to follow a strict vegetarian diet (and much less make a small child follow it) unless you have a good handle on nutrition principles. Strict vegetarians should always take B_{12} supplements and this is especially true during pregnancy and breastfeeding. There is a wealth of information on the Internet on reputable vegetarian sites.[39,40]

Macrobiotic diets are progressive; as they advance toward "perfection", they are more restrictive. It is considered to be an inadequate diet for children, and also for pregnant or breastfeeding mothers. There have been severe cases of B_{12} deficiency in breastfed babies whose mothers were following macrobiotic or very strict vegetarian diets (without milk or eggs).

Won't he be missing some nutrients?

No. If you offer an adequate diet, your child will get what he needs, no matter how little he eats.

Of course, if his diet consists of potato chips and sweets, he might be missing something, but your baby is too young to go to the store and buy these things; he can only eat what his parents offer. (See my comments about iron on page 119)

Why won't he try new things?

My son is almost three and I am very concerned because he has never been one to try new things.

In this world there are many plants and some animals that are poisonous. One of the protective mechanisms that we animals possess is a preference for known foods and an initial rejection of new foods.

He is fifteen months old. He used to want to try everything, but lately he only eats things he has tasted before. I can't even get anything new to come to his mouth.

What better protection than to eat what your parents eat? It has been proven that animals taste through their mother's milk the flavours of the foods that the mother ingests. So, the sheep that get their mother's milk prefer to eat the same kind of grass that their mothers ate, while the sheep that are fed artificially show no such preferences. Although we've not conducted a similar experiment, we suppose that the same holds true in humans. This might be one of the reasons why breastfed babies seem to reject baby foods: they don't like vanilla-flavoured cereal, or mixed strained fruit because these are not foods their mothers eat. On the other hand they often accept (and beg for) bites off their mothers' plate.

Therefore, rejecting new foods is totally normal for children, especially if they have not tasted the flavour through their mother's milk. You don't have to make them eat a new food (they would reject it) but it is also not necessary to remove said food from the family diet. It has been shown that if children are offered a food regularly (without forcing!) and if they see their parents eating it many times, they end up accepting it (though not always, of course).

Shouldn't he get used to eating everything?

When was the last time you went to a wedding banquet? Do you remember the menu?

In many cases, the caterer prepares a separate menu for the children. While the adults feast on elaborate and exotic salads or seafood with creative sauces, the children have their own "children's menu", almost always consisting of some sort of familiar foods like pasta or fried chicken with French fries. I have never seen any one of the adults (not even the younger adults) tell a waiter: "I don't like this, could you bring me a kids' meal?"

Incidentally, children often eat very well at these parties, since no one is making them eat. You will also see adults eating foods they have never tasted before, often saying how wonderful everything is.

After seeing thousands of children and adults eat, professional caterers know that it is impossible to make a child eat "everything". They also know that adults like to try new foods even if they were raised on macaroni.

Follow their example and don't worry about it. Your child will eat all sorts of things (at least the things you have at home) when he reaches a certain age. Meanwhile, the best way to get a child to never eat a certain food is to make him eat it.

By the way, many children are willing to eat a wide range of foods when they are about two years old, and then after that they become picky eaters. Between the ages of four or five and adolescence, some children seem to always want the same things: rice, macaroni, French fries, bread, chocolate milk, over and over.

Do you eat everything? In every culture there are foods that are considered edible and others that are not. I would never eat certain things that are considered edible in my country, such as snails or pigs' feet; much less ants and filet of dog, which are considered normal food in other countries. If I were invited to eat some of these foods, my hosts would just have to think I was not raised well since I don't eat everything.

What if my baby were born with a low weight?

I am the mother of a five-month-old baby who was born by induction at 36 weeks due to intrauterine growth retardation. She weighed 1.950 kg (4 lbs 4.5 oz) at birth and currently weighs 5.800 kg (12 lbs 12 oz).

The baby used to eat marvellously, asking for more at each feeding. It almost alarmed me to see how quickly she would finish her bottles. But as soon as she turned two months, she started leaving a little more at each feeding. She is still doing that. She eats four times a day taking in a total of 480 ml (16 oz) of milk per twenty-four hours. I put two scoops of cereal in each bottle.

Intrauterine growth retardation is often due to a specific problem, for example, a placenta that does not nourish the fetus normally. That is why this mother was induced: so that her daughter could gain weight. And that is what she did. She had "back hunger" and ate like a piggy until her weight normalized. This is another brilliant example illustrating how children eat what they need. Once she reached her mark, she started eating normally (to the despair of her mother, Silvia, who did not expect the change.)

Not all children born at low weight show this swift recovery. Depending on the cause of the problem, it is possible that they may still eat very little and grow slowly for years.

Premature or underweight children have fewer reserves of iron, and may need iron drops. Consult your doctor.

Shouldn't I put him on a schedule?

Are you on a schedule? Do you eat breakfast, lunch and dinner at the same time on Sunday as well as on Wednesday? When you want to watch the big game or an interesting movie on television, do you not eat earlier or later? What if you go out to the movies or eat out?

Meal schedules are one of the most interesting myths of our culture. In reality, no one follows a rigid eating schedule. It is not necessary to eat at certain times to stay healthy, nor to aid digestion. This "popular wisdom" contradicts itself: for example, some say it is dangerous to go to sleep on a full stomach, without having time to digest food properly, while others recommend precisely that you fill your baby up with a big meal just before bed so he will sleep through the night.

It is only when we are employed that we are made to adapt and eat before or after work. This is the same reason your child will follow a schedule as soon as he goes to school. He will drink his milk before leaving the house, have a snack at recess, eat lunch after morning class, and have an afternoon snack upon returning home. Or do you think that, if you don't give him his baby food at a set time, your child's "rhythm" will be so altered that at twelve years old he'll have to take a container of macaroni with him to eat during the maths class?

It is also not necessary to feed him always in the same place or using the same routine. Your child will eat some meals in his high chair, others on your lap. He will eat some foods with his fingers, others with a spoon. He will eat sometimes at home and at other times at grandma's. He will sometimes even eat while walking down the street.

If it were really necessary (which it is not) to teach one- and two-year-olds to follow adult social norms, then what we should teach them is not to follow a schedule. Can you imagine that at twelve years old, when your child is visiting grandmother and lunch is not ready until 1:30 pm, he might start crying at 12:00 noon saying: "I'm hungry, I'm hungry, I'm hungry", because as a baby you always fed him at 12:00 noon? How would you like to have a child who acts that way?

Is it bad to eat between meals?

This is simply an extension of the previous myth. Food is food, no matter when you eat it.

Animals don't have set mealtimes. Large carnivores eat huge "meals" widely spaced; but not at set times, only when they have a successful hunt. Herbivores and insectivores eat all day, whenever they find something to put in their mouth, until they are full.

In reality, several scientific studies indicate that eating small amounts of food frequently throughout the day is probably better for humans than eating the large, widely spaced meals that we commonly eat.[2] Laboratory rats that are fed large amounts of food only a few times a day accumulate more body fat than those that are allowed to eat all day, even if they consume the same amount of calories. They also produce more cholesterol and their stomach becomes abnormally enlarged. In other words, their system responds to the danger of not having food when needed by increasing its capacity to store food during the times of abundance.

In humans, those who eat only at set times (few meals, but in abundance) have higher cholesterol and lower glucose tolerance than those who "snack" (eating small, frequent meals). This is why diabetics are told to eat five or six times a day.

For this same reason, to try to get a baby to "sleep through the night" without waking to eat seems as though it might be a bad idea for his metabolism.[2] Theoretically, although the child could eat more during the day and then fast all night, it is probably better that he eats frequently. Breastfeeding during the night should therefore not be considered a "bad habit", but a need.

How long can a baby go without eating?

My question is: at what age should I stop waking my eight-month-old for feedings? The doctor has told me not to let more than five hours elapse without feeding her so that her blood glucose doesn't go down too much.

Newborns lose weight, and the less they nurse, the more weight they lose. Sometimes they fall into a vicious cycle: they lose so much weight that they are too weak to cry, and since they don't cry, mother doesn't feed them. Therefore, it is sensible to try to breastfeed a newly born baby at least every four hours, even if he doesn't ask to be fed. It might be smart to offer a child of any age frequent feedings if he is sick or losing weight, but never to force him.

However, there is no need to wake up to feed a healthy child who is consistently gaining weight, whether at eight months or two weeks, unless the mother needs to feed the baby because her breasts are so full or because she is about to go out, for example.

Should I wait between feeding and swimming or a bath?

There is no such thing as disruption of digestion, known among many people of Hispanic origin as "corte de digestión". Nothing happens if you get wet after eating.

Each summer the media in Spain report that a swimmer died due to "corte de digestión". That is not true. He drowned. Perhaps, it is true that some people do feel heavy and fatigued after eating a large meal, and this might promote an accident if they should swim too far from shore. But there is no danger at the edge of the water, and even less in a bathtub. You can bathe your child right after eating.

Why does he eat at school but not at home?

Children often behave "better" for strangers than for their parents. We cannot hold back our surprise when a teacher assures us that at school our child picks up the toys or puts on his jacket by himself. Those green with envy would say that our children are manipulating us; but do not be fooled. In reality this just shows they love us.

To begin with, we all do this. Don't you put up with aggravation from your boss that you'd never put up with from your husband? It is a matter of trust, and we hope our children can tell the difference between home and school!

And you, dear father and reader, where did you obey more, where did you complain more? Where did you make your bed, fold your clothes better, sweep and clean up better? At home or in the military? Would you like to go back to boot camp? Did you love your sergeant more than your mother?

Going back to food, we must differentiate between the amount of food eaten and manners (if he eats quickly, without playing, without making a mess or getting out of his seat…). It makes sense that your child eats with better manners at school, where he feels watched, than at home, where he feels loved and safe. But the amount of food, what he does or does not eat, is a different issue and this difference usually stems from a very simple reason: his carers do not make him eat at school or day care.

We should never force a child to eat for several reasons; one of them is that the more you try to force the issue, the less the child eats. At day care, even if the carers wanted to, they can't force children to eat. Typically there is one worker per ten children. There is not enough time to beg for two hours or to do "the airplane"; he who is quick, eats. And of course, most children make it snappy.

There are exceptions. Some children eat even less at school than at home. In such cases, normally it's because they are forced more at school. It is unbelievable to me that some mentally unstable people do find the time to force children to eat. Devoid of the love that moderates the behaviour of mothers, these people sometimes behave with unspeakable cruelty. We have seen children who have been forced to eat their vomit. Never ignore your child's protests; a child who is terrified of school may have good reason.

If your child is the victim of ill treatment, regarding food or any other topic, be quick to get him to safety and report the incident to the authorities. If he is made to eat, but without resorting to extremes, try to reason with those responsible at school or day care centre to convince them not to force him. If logical arguments are not enough, don't hesitate to use literary licence such as: "Antonio's stomach doesn't close properly and the doctor has told us to never force him to eat because he could aspirate." This should be enough to command reasonable respect.

The same goes for children who feel a particular revulsion for any particular food. A few years ago there was a terrible incident in a Spanish hospital. A young child, allergic to dairy products and hospitalized for another reason, died after being given yogurt. The allergy had not been noted in the clinical history but the child, in spite of his young age, had been taught by his parents to refuse any dairy product. Someone on the staff ignored his refusal and force-fed him a yogurt.

I can just imagine this. The child screaming, crying, closing his mouth, trying to explain he doesn't eat yogurt, and in fact, must not. Perhaps one of the staff sees this and says: "This child is just spoiled, his mother just lets him get away with it, and he just takes advantage. Bring the yogurt here and I'll show you how he eats it."

This case should be enough to make sure that no one would ever dare to make a child eat at school or in a hospital. Unfortunately, although the event was in the news for quite a while, it seems that everyone has forgotten it now. I am not implying that all children who refuse a certain food have an allergy or are in real danger, but they have their reasons and those reasons deserve our respect. If you can't obtain this respect at the school through reasonable means, don't hesitate to say that your child has an allergy.

Should we allow him to get away with it?

In life it is common for two people to have differing opinions. Our children must learn to act appropriately in these cases. They must learn to defend their opinions with reasonable arguments, and to listen with respect to the arguments and opinions of others, concede when someone is right, and expect respect when reason is on their side. They also need to learn to yield with dignity and to come to satisfactory compromises.

Unfortunately many "experts" in parenting (and few fields have such a large panel of experts, from those who write books to the ones we meet in the elevator) insist that children need to be raised with a firm hand and, if you yield your authority once, you have lost it for good. They state that rules should be few but unbreakable (another version prefers many rules, but just as immutable), that to give a child what he asks for when he is crying and screaming is "rewarding him" and therefore you are encouraging him to cry and yell even more the next time.

Why should only parents be endowed with this absolute power? We would hope employers listen to their workers' grievances. We hope that the laws will not proceed from the will of a tyrant, but from a democratic consensus. Even before a judge, it is possible to present appeals and arguments. Do the judges fear a loss of authority if the defendant "gets away with it"?

We must ask ourselves what kind of children we want to raise: responsible, caring, and able to engage in dialogue, sure of themselves and having firm convictions? Or are we looking for obedient and obsequious adults? According to our answer we must then ask if we can afford not to have our children "get away with it", especially when they are in the right.

Why does my child eat less than my neighbour's child?

So what if the neighbour's child eats more? Is he by chance more adorable than yours? Or smarter? Well then, let his mother enjoy the satisfaction of winning on the food issue.

There are many reasons why some children eat more or less than others. Of course, age, size, rate of growth, and physical activity are all important. But there are also intrinsic metabolic factors in each case. We all know people who "live on air" and others who "eat everything in sight".

While many of our neighbours' children may eat more, there are also some who eat less. But sometimes there is a misunderstanding: what do you call eating little, and what does the neighbour consider eating a lot?

A friend of ours was complaining bitterly about how little her son ate. "He always leaves more than half his plate. Does your child eat well?" she would ask us anxiously. "Well, yes," we would respond. "Does he finish his plate?" "Yes, he usually does." She seemed so worried, convinced that her son was the only child in the world who did not eat. We sometimes wished we could tell a little white lie just to make her feel better. (In fact, we've started to respond to these questions by saying: "No, he doesn't eat a thing, but he's strong and healthy and that is what matters!")

One summer we went on vacation together. At mealtime our friend stared in amazement at the plate of food we gave our child. "Is that all you're going to give him?" "Well, yes." "Will it be enough?" "Sure. If we give him more, he wouldn't be able to finish it." Her face changed, much as the ancient Greek Achimedes' face must have changed when he jumped out of the bath shouting, "Eureka!". She ran to empty her son's plate (she had given him twice as much as we had given our child!). Her son (of course) ate everything; she never again had problems with food.

Why won't he eat foods that he used to like?

Children's preferences change with time. It is not rare for a baby who was a great fan of bananas to subtly change his allegiance over to apples; or for Miguelito who used to love to drink milk, to refuse to touch it for a year, and then suddenly want it again . . . or not.

When will he learn to eat alone?

Before a year, and sometimes before their first taste of food, children often try to get food into their mouths. This is not necessarily the same as eating alone, because they probably don't want mother to leave; but prefer for her to watch and praise their ability to pick up peas with their fingers. If you let them practice, they will soon eat perfectly, with their fingers or a spoon, including drinking "solo" from a cup.

If we reject these first bursts of autonomy because of our haste or in order to get him to eat more, it is easy for the baby to lose interest in the topic; by eighteen months he may not even show any interest in self-feeding, as it's now become so easy for him to have someone else put food into his mouth.

There is nothing wrong with teaching a child to only eat when an adult feeds him, as long as you are willing to keep doing it for years without grumbling. What is not fair is to teach him to only eat when an adult feeds him and then to complain because he won't eat by himself.

In any case, "to feed him" should never be the same as "to make him eat". Whether he eats by himself or you feed him, the plate should be taken away when your child says (or uses his gestures to say): "I'm finished."

Frequently a baby (or toddler) who had been eating independently suddenly asks to be fed. He may feel sick, jealous, or simply want to pretend to be little. It's a small indulgence that is not harmful. Accept it as a sign of love and don't allow wicked people to tell you that your child "is manipulating you" or "is regressing". On the contrary, this is totally normal behaviour, similar to that descibed by the child psychiatrist, John Bowlby:[41]

> This is true even in the bird world. Young finches quite capable of feeding themselves will at once start begging for food in an infantile way if they catch sight of their parents.

How many calories does my child need?

If we've talked about calories in this book, it has been just by way of example. I had to dig out these facts from books that I had never looked at before, not as a parent nor as a paediatrician. Knowing the caloric needs of a child or of an adult may be helpful for scientists and researchers or in very special cases, as for patients in a coma who must be fed with a tube. But such caloric facts are not helpful when feeding a healthy child.

First of all, children's needs, just like adults' needs, are highly variable. They change depending on the age and weight of the child, but even children of the same age and weight can ingest very different amounts. Day to day needs also vary. Why do you need to know that your daughter needs between 84.2 and 120.8 kcal per 1 kg (2.2 lbs) of weight per day? (A huge difference of almost 50 percent. This is actual data for artificially fed baby girls between days 50 and 83).[2] Your baby's real needs could fall anywhere in that wide range, even a bit below or above it. On the other hand, your daughter knows exactly what she needs.

Secondly, our understanding of children's needs keeps changing. As mentioned above, there are new studies, more precise ones, about the caloric needs of children. The numbers I just gave you: between 84.2 and 120.8 kcal per day are outdated and have been updated. According to Butte,[4] artificially fed three-month-old baby girls (in other words, ninety days old) need between 59.7 and 117 kcal/kg per day. The mean has been lowered and the range has expanded; we recognize that some children eat more than twice as much as others, even those who are the same age and weight.

It is hard to compare different authors' recommendations since they often refer to different age ranges. Dewey and Brown[42] have made the necessary calculations in order to be able to make fair comparisons. Just as an amusing aside, in 1985, the WHO recommended that children (both genders) from twelve to twenty-three months should eat 1170 kcal per day; while Butte, in 2000,[4] estimated that 894 kcal were needed, a 24 percent reduction. Between nine and eleven months, the recommended caloric intake decreased by 28 percent. A quarter of the dietary "needs" have been wiped off the map in fifteen short years. And these are numbers from 1985 that the first edition of this book referred to as "newer", as opposed to the "older" ones that were higher still. You might have a book at home that recommends exactly what amount of food to feed your child based on his age, but the recommendations may be based on nearly "prehistoric" data.

Thirdly, even if it were possible (which it is not) to know exactly how many calories your baby needs, you wouldn't be able to know if she'd ingested this amount or not. You may know how many calories are in a yogurt or a custard because you can read the label and commercial products are always the same. But, how many calories are in a plate of pasta? It will depend on how much sauce you put on and if that sauce has more or less oil, and whether or not you add Parmesan cheese. Scientists use very elaborate methods to measure caloric intake in their experiments; trying to do this at home is diet-fiction.

Healthy feeding behaviours are guided by internal cues (hunger and satiety), not external ones (pressures, promises, punishments and publicity). Experts believe that many of the problems in adolescence and adult life, such as obsessive dieting and compulsive eating, stem from what was learned in infancy; to eat according to external cues.[14] Give your child the gift of a lifetime: let him learn to eat according to his own needs, not according to some chart.

Talk is cheap; I'd like to see what Doctor González would do if his children refused to eat like mine.

You are too late, I'm afraid. My children are already grown. Yes, they did grow, even though they did not eat. Why do you think I know that a child can get up and skip breakfast, or go to bed without dinner, or go all day on only one yogurt and two crackers? Why do you think that I know that some stop eating at a year and others refuse solids until ten months? How do you think I found out that they could go for a year without tasting milk, or bananas? Why do you think I insist that all this is normal?

For the same reasons I know that, if you show respect and don't make them eat, they eat what they need and grow happy and healthy.

I don't speak from hearsay. I have been there, done that.

Appendix
A bit of history

"My child won't eat" is such a common and anxiety-filled complaint that one is tempted to think that it is an ancient concern for humankind, ever existent, like fear of the dark or of wolves. Years ago, I too thought that this fear that mothers expressed of their baby not eating had a long history stemming from the time when lack of appetite was the first symptom of tuberculosis or another (then) incurable disease, the harbinger of death.

However, after reading some old books, I started to have my doubts. Is it possible that children who "don't eat" are a relatively new phenomenon?

In the time of Dr. Ulecia y Cardona, who in 1906 published *Arte de criar a los niños* (*The Art of Raising Children*),[43] it would seem that mothers did not complain to the paediatrician about their babies not eating. On the contrary, they were proud of their healthy appetites, much to the doctor's concern:

> How often we hear parents boast totally satisfied about their child's appetite saying: "You should see how well he eats; he eats everything . . . !"
>
> And how many, after a time, do we hear lamenting the loss of this child saying: "Poor thing! He was eating everything when he died." They do not understand, unfortunately, that it was precisely this that caused the baby's demise more than anything else.

The greatest fear among infant nutrition experts of that time (Dr. Ulecia studied in Paris with Dr. Budin, one of the greatest paediatricians of his time) was precisely excess feeding, "an unpardonable crime".

The introduction of solids took place very cautiously. Until twelve months old, ten at the earliest, Dr. Ulecia recommends exclusive breastfeeding. At this age you could start offering a clear gruel made with water and flour followed by breastfeeding.

A full day's intake for a one-year-old was as follows:

8:00 am – 9:00 am: breastfeed.

Noon: gruel made with flour . . . not to be made with broth, *no matter how pure, because fats are not good* for babies in their first months.

These gruels must be *very thin at first*, then a little thicker with time . . . I do not recommend gruel made with milk; I prefer them to be made with water, and after the gruel, breastfeed for dessert.

4:00 pm: breastfeed.

7:00 pm: 130 g [4.6 oz] milk.

11:00 pm: breastfeed.

After midnight – same as last month, only one feeding at the breast.

At around thirteen to fourteen months, Dr. Ulecia recommends adding an egg yolk to the morning gruel, and adding another feeding of plain gruel in the afternoon. At fifteen months, he suggests adding egg yolk to both gruels. At sixteen or eighteen months, broth, legumes, and crackers were added (once a day). At twenty or twenty-one months, breastfeeding was suspended, even at night, and crackers were allowed three times a day. At twenty-two to twenty-four months, chocolate, fish and brains were added.

At three years old, whole egg was introduced and chicken croquettes made according to a special recipe. The amount of fish is specified as "the size of a Spanish dollar or a bit more" (Spanish dollars at the time measured 37 mm or 1.5 in). Three 100 g (3.5 oz) servings of milk were given per day (less than half a cup!).

At three-and-a-half, fruit was introduced: "They may tolerate a few grapes." The child got milk (130 to 150 g, or 4.6 to 5.2 oz) twice a day.

Vegetables were introduced when the child turned four, but "only a little", the same as veal; also "Moderate quantities of fruit, except for cantaloupe, watermelon, and peaches . . ." and never in the evening.

Do you now understand why children did eat back then? Can you see that, had you lived at that time, you would have gotten a good tongue lashing from Dr. Ulecia when he heard everything your darling angel does eat? Fruit, vegetables, meat and fish before one year, glassfuls of milk . . . you are going to kill him! (And you would have had to pay ten pesetas for the visit, which was a small fortune.) Remember this the next time your baby does not want fruit: his great-great-grandfather did not taste fruit until three years old!

The problem of the "child who won't eat" stems from a difference between what the child eats and what his mother expects him to eat. It is likely that children have always eaten, more or less, the same. But the amount that mothers expected them to eat (at least those mothers who went to a doctor or read books) has drastically changed in the last century. Today, if our daughter takes three bites of apple we are in a panic because we've been led to believe that she should have eaten half the apple, half a pear, half a banana, and half an orange with some crackers. Our great-grandmother also ate only three bites of an apple, but our great-great-grandmother wouldn't dare tell the doctor.

We have been told that it is important to get children used to a variety of foods while they are young, otherwise they will refuse them later and will become picky eaters. This is untrue. Our great grandparents didn't eat "regular food" until they were five and somehow adapted perfectly to an adult diet: nothing less than the famous Mediterranean diet, without artificial food colourings or preservatives. Could it be that fruits, vegetables, and legumes were like a long-awaited treat 100 years ago, and now we have made them into a dreaded threat?

Twenty years later, in 1927, Dr. Puig y Roig,[44] in his book *Puericultura* (*Child Rearing*), does not even mention the existence of children who won't eat. He recommends the first food (a bread and garlic soup) at six or eight months. At one year, a baby's diet would be:

6:00 am: breastfeed.
9:00 am: breastfeed.
12:00 noon: salty soup.
4:00 pm: breastfeed.
7:00 pm: sweet gruel.
11:00 pm: breastfeed.

Salty soup is made of only bread, salt and garlic. Sweet gruel is made with oat or rice flour and may have milk. Unfortunately, Dr. Puig's work concentrates on the first year with very vague indications regarding the introduction of other foods.

We are able to find all the details in the work of his colleague and fellow citizen, Dr. S. Goday,[45] who a year later published *Alimentació del nen durant la primera infància* (*Feeding During the First Year of Infancy*) (1928), the only book quoted here that is not directed at mothers, but at doctors. It does not mention lack of appetite or children who "don't eat". It also recommends the first food to be a thin gruel of flour and water at eight months; and at one year (between ten and fifteen months) it recommends the following diet:

Two servings of gruel made of flour [flour and water] and four nursings (or four cups of milk with sugar). After one year an egg yolk can be added to the gruel once a day. Instead of these, a gruel made with milk [milk and flour] may also be substituted.

Between fifteen and eighteen months mashed potatoes, eggs, and pastas were introduced; between eighteen and twenty-four months, meats and fish.

Pureed vegetables, such as spinach, can be given in small quantity. They are not very nutritious . . .

169

Fruit could be given from eighteen months, but only cooked fruit, such as compote or preserves. Only during the third year did Goday authorize the use of fresh fruit in small quantities.

Dr. Goday's recommendations are far removed from today's, although Dr. Ulecia was probably having fits (the old man was no doubt thinking: "Vegetables before two years? At least it's only a little!").

Dr. Roig y Raventós, in the 1932, fourth edition of his *Nocions de puericultura* (*Principles on Child Rearing*)[46] has similar recommendations. First food (a small amount of garlic and bread soup, followed by breastfeeding) was given at eight, or better yet, ten months. The diet of the one-year-old has barely changed:

7:00 am:	breastfeed.
10:00 am:	bottle.
1:00 pm:	salty soup and breastfeed.
4:00 pm:	breastfeed.
7:00 pm:	sweet gruel and breastfeed.
10:00 pm:	breastfeed.

The salty soup contained water, bread, and garlic.

At eighteen months you could start bread with butter, egg yolk, tomato, grape and orange juice, pasta and legumes. Fish was given at two-and-a-half years, and chicken at age three.

For Dr. Roig, excess feeding remained the chief danger:

Most childhood illnesses stem from overfeeding.

Although still much less than current recommendations, in the 1920s and 1930s feeding started earlier and in bigger amounts than at the turn of the century. Why was that? How did this affect children's appetite? Dr. Roig does not speak about lack of appetite in 1932, but it might be that the conflict was just brewing. Sooner or later, if recommendations keep increasing, a certain number of children will be unable to eat everything that is recommended.

By 1936, in the fifth edition of his book,[47] Dr. Roig had made some modifications. Solids creep in earlier. The phrase:

At the end of the second six months, it is good for the baby to taste salty food. (1932)

has been replaced with:

In the second six months, it is good for the baby to taste salty food. (1936)

Raw fruit juice is also introduced starting at four months, in order to prevent scurvy:

Scurvy presents itself in children raised on sterilized, modified milks, which chemistry has profaned to the point of destroying the few vitamins they contain in an attempt to make them similar to mother's milk.

As the amount of solids increase, the amount of children who are unable to eat everything also increases. In 1936 we see the conflict arise. It comes to light when Dr. Roig adds three chapters to his book, three chapters dedicated to low weight, rickets and lack of appetite. This last topic takes up two pages: "Lack of appetite in children is one of the most frequent family concerns."

So here we have the full picture: children who don't eat and worried mothers! However, in those days there was a group of mothers (which seem extinct nowadays) who were as strange to Dr. Roig as they were threatening: those mothers who were not worried. Those who still defended the right of their child to refuse food, thereby rejecting the doctor's expert recommendations:

One scene that sadly is repeated in the doctor's office is the following: after finding an adequate regime for the clinical case at hand and reading it to the family, sometimes even before finishing the reading, the mother, in front of her child, interrupts the physician to say: "He will never eat all the food you are recommending!" The child knows from that moment that he has in his mother a defender of his stubborn food refusal. This mother is ignorant and unworthy of caring for a child. . . . Never should a superior authority, much less a doctor, be discredited in front of a child.

Fortunately modern-day doctors do not consider themselves superior to a mother, nor do they think that any mother who does not unquestionably obey her doctor's recommendations is "unworthy of caring for a child".

At other times, the mother appears to be blamed for showing too much affection:

It is also sadly frequent that a lack of appetite, as well as vomiting in school age children, is present in children surrounded by over-concentrated intimate affection . . . Vomiting is the end of the battle that happens daily with children who present nervous lack of appetite.

Lastly, the mother might simply be mistaken:

There also exists an imagined lack of appetite. Children eat well, but their mothers, with no scientific basis, imagine that their children do not eat enough, and a daily useless battle ensues.

What is blatantly lacking is mention of the child who refuses to eat because he does not need the amount of food that his doctor had prescribed. Instead of reviewing their theories in light of the failure of their application, nutrition experts at that time push through full steam ahead. In his last edition, written in 1947, Dr. Roig[48] includes some drastic changes.

The first food (garlic soup) is offered earlier. The recommend-ation moves from eight or ten months, to six months. The menu for the one-year-old child is the same as in 1932, although the times have changed without explanation (now they are 6:00 am, 9:00 am, 12:00 noon, 4:00 pm, 9:00 pm and midnight). However, the "salty soup" of 1932 that had contained only bread and garlic, in 1947 includes cheese, chicken, or fish:

Some children at around seven or eight months can tolerate half an egg yolk or a teaspoon of grated cheese or a teaspoon of butter that must be boiled for two minutes, or even a teaspoon of pureed liver (boiled and strained). Offer a different food each day.

The first "training" bottle is also offered earlier: at six months versus ten months. Terrible consequences are threatened for children who do not consume the prescribed food at the prescribed times. Curiously enough, ages are moved ahead by six months, and children who were perfectly fine yesterday will waste away today without any explanation for the change in recommendations:

> It is necessary that by the end of the first year, the child eat more than just breast milk. Breast milk is low in iron and if the child is raised only on this lacteal secretion, he will become white and flabby. These are "curd babies" (1936).
> It is necessary that by the end of the first semester (six months), the child eat more than just breast milk. Breast milk is low in iron and if the child is raised only on this lacteal secretion, he will become white and flabby. These are "cream babies" (1947).

For Dr. R. Ramos, who in 1941[49] published the first edition of his book *Puericultura* (*Child Rearing*), with the second edition in 1949, the problem of "the child who won't eat" does not seem to be given much importance. The book spends ample space on the education and discipline of infants and young children, but he only devotes two paragraphs to the subject of food:

> When a child that usually eats well suddenly stops eating, the mother must not insist or force him to eat, on the contrary, let her feed the child only mineral water, juice, or tea for a few hours, which should be enough to overcome this state.

However, the recognition that some children may not need as much food does not make him revise his general recommendations. Juice at three months, cereals at four, strained vegetables at five, strained fruits at five-and-a-half months, crackers at six, egg yolk at seven, liver at eight . . . By ten months the diet is certainly ample, with interesting changes between 1941 and 1949.

In 1941, Dr. Ramos recommends the following for children between the ages of nine and twelve months:

6:00 am: first nursing.
9:00 am: strained fruit with crackers.
12:00 pm: strained vegetables with liver. Second nursing.
4:00 pm: gruel with strained egg yolk. (At one year, one yolk). Third nursing.
8:00 pm: wheat, tapioca, or oatmeal gruel. Juice or breastfeeding.
11:00 pm: gruel. Fourth or fifth nursing.
Two crackers per day or a small piece of bread.

While in 1949 he recommends, for children between ten and twelve months:

7:00 am: first nursing.
10:00 am: 150 g [5.2 oz] gruel with a heaping teaspoon of flour or maize meal. Three teaspoons of egg yolk, three times per week that will increase until one whole yolk is eaten by one year, three times per week. Second nursing.
2:00 pm: three teaspoons of mixed strained vegetables mixed with one teaspoon (ten months) or two teaspoons (at one year) of potato. Three teaspoons of liver on the three days that egg is not given. A bit of boiled or mineral water. Strained fruit.
6:00 pm: 150 g [5.2 oz] of gruel with a heaping teaspoon of flour or maize meal. Third nursing. (Wean at one year.)
10:00 pm: from five to eight tablespoons of soup (from 75 to 120 cc). Fourth nursing.

Some significant changes were made in only eight years and by the very same author. On the one hand, we see a reduction from six to only five meals. On the other hand, more paediatrician control is emphasized; grams, cubic centimetres, days of the week to feed egg yolk and liver are specified. (No, there was no freedom about that in the first edition. This is only the summary chart, and the book has previously explained these details over several pages. The difference is in emphasis: in 1949, Dr. Ramos considers the details important enough to repeat them in the summary charts.)

Will children eat all this? There are reasons to doubt it.

For Dr. Blancafort, who published his book *Puericultura actual* (*Modern Child Rearing*) in 1979,[50] the topic of children who didn't eat is an important one: "A frequent cause of mother-child problems", he writes. In the first section of his chapter, "Most Frequent Digestive Alterations in Children", he spends six pages on the topic, with descriptions the same as any modern-day doctor would make:

> Lack of appetite or anorexia . . . is one of the most frequent reasons for worried mothers to visit the paediatrician. The mother believes that if the situation were to continue, her child will starve to death . . . . It should be considered a passing phase, not abnormal for many children . . . . In general, this problem of lack of appetite is not an issue until after the first birthday.

The treatment Dr. Blancafort recommends is very similar to what is explained in this book: do not force the child, don't distract, and don't threaten. Do not give medication and recognize that he does not need to eat as much. But this compassionate attitude does not stop him from starting solids even earlier than before, starting at three months and not slowly, but abruptly: from day one, two servings of flour and milk gruel, and one serving of fruit. At four months, vegetables. Egg yolk and liver at six months (but sometimes at four).

The food lists no longer include breastfeeding for children of ten to twelve months. And what is most surprising, they also do not mention bottles. The 1970s marked the triumph of "solids":

> Breakfast: sweet gruel that can be accompanied with crackers or bread.
> Lunch: soup or strained vegetables or potatoes with added

meat, liver, or brains, etc. Fruit for dessert, or some cheese.

Afternoon snack: strained fruit or fruit yogurt or crackers.

Dinner: sweet gruel with egg yolk or soup with egg yolk, ham, fish, or one béchamel (a white sauce made with milk, flour, and butter).

At one year, dried legumes, fruits, sauces, candies, cakes and cocoa were introduced. No wonder Dr. Blancafort had to write six whole pages on the topic of lack of appetite!

This does not pretend to be an exhaustive historical analysis, I have not systematically searched all the literature regarding this topic. But it would seem that the child who "won't eat", as a concern for mothers and a reason for doctors' visits, was born in the 1930s and gradually spread following the changing recommendations for infant and young child feeding.

It seems that child feeding has changed throughout the last century almost as much as the length of skirts or the widths of ties. Each new generation of doctors has recommended a totally different diet from the previous generation (in other words, different from what they learned in medical school and very different from what they ate as infants). Each doctor also changed his recommendations as his career progressed. Each generation of paediatricians has encountered the challenge of "teaching" new scientific discoveries to mothers, fighting the grandmothers' advice that followed thirty-year-old medical norms. These poor mothers and grandmothers who were only repeating what another doctor had said, or what they found in a book, are labelled as ignorant in infant nutrition. Not one author takes the time to talk about the old diets in order to explain the differences and the reason for changes. Instead, each author recommends diets recently invented, as if he were preaching the Ten Commandments, and demands instant obedience.

Today's doctors, who are now recommending that mothers wait until six months to start solids, are faced with mothers and especially grandmothers who were used to the early introduction of solids in the 1970s. ("What do you mean just breastfeeding?

He should be eating three times a day by now!") Seventy years ago, the problem was exactly the opposite, and Dr. José Muñoz,[51] author of the book *Madre . . . cría a tu hijo!* (*Mother, Nurse Your Child!*) (1941), speaks critically of grandmother's interference in this imaginary dialogue:

> "What are you doing? Starting solids already?" . . .
> "The doctor has ordered it, and since I am under his care, I want to follow his instructions faithfully."
> "I don't know what to say," answers grandmother, "In my day we loved our children more; I had five and I gave them nothing but breast milk for 26 months. It's all about trends. How times have changed! Nowadays, you want to do everything in a hurry, quickly . . . let baby walk quickly, let him talk quickly, let him eat quickly . . . ."

Notice the phrase, "follow his instructions faithfully". Obedience becomes the supreme virtue. In this dialogue, the mother seems stiff, like a robot, giving stereotypical answers while the grandmother, on the other hand, lives and thinks and has personal opinions based on her experience. Even if the grandmother was advocating a totally different view, such as recommending the first solid food at two months, you can't help but sympathize with her. However, Dr. Muñoz thought that with this dialogue he was praising the mother and making the grandmother look foolish. In that way he helped mothers to disregard the opinions of their own mothers and listen to him instead. Really, how times have changed!

It would be absurd to think, however, that child feeding changes simply because of fashion or trends. We are talking about true nutrition experts who were up-to-date in all the scientific advances of their time. Perhaps they were mistaken (it is hard to believe that they were all right, since they made such divergent recommendations), but certainly there had to be a reason for these sweeping changes

I believe the reason was artificial feeding. In 1906 practically every child was breastfed by his mother or a wet nurse. (Dr.

Ulecia offered wet nurse examinations for 15 pesetas – a very high fee.) Some children were artificially fed, mostly on mixtures of cow's milk and sugar with disastrous consequences, as you may well imagine. Babies do not have the ability to easily digest and metabolize the excess proteins and mineral salts in cow's milk and thus it became essential to strictly limit how much they were getting. This is where the great concern over strict schedules and overfeeding was born.

Unfortunately, experts started to think that those schedules, perhaps necessary for babies who were drinking cow's milk, would also be beneficial for breastfed infants. Even when the percentage of babies being artificially fed was low, doctors soon had more experience with bottle-fed babies simply because they were sicker and came to see them more often. In those times, the poor did not go to the doctor, even if they were sick, much less if they were healthy (to take a child to the doctor for a "well baby checkup" was unthinkable). It is hard to fathom today (unless you are acquainted with Third World countries, where the situation remains the same) the terrible mortality that artificial feeding brought about in those times. Dr. Ulecia quotes another expert on this topic, Dr. Variot from France:

> Mothers who withhold the breast from their children, especially in the early months, feeding them from birth exclusively with artificial foods, expose them to a greater risk of death than what a soldier undergoes in the field of battle.

Babies who breastfed for one year grew without problems, since mother's milk contains all the necessary vitamins and nutrients; for the few babies who drank whole cow's milk, the concern was not to overload the digestive tract. But things deteriorated rapidly. Twenty years later, Dr. Roig complained that it was harder to find a good wet nurse, and his books are full of ads for formula.

In the 1930s, babies drank artificial baby milks that had reduced protein, but also reduced vitamins due to processing and sterilizing. Now they needed other foods, especially fruits, vegetables and liver to avoid scurvy and other vitamin deficiencies;

cereals and other home-cooked foods to reduce the need for costly artificial baby milk. (Poorer mothers would once again use whole cow's milk, probably without sterilizing it. This was hard for baby to digest and sometimes laden with tuberculosis.)

Excessive enthusiasm led to food recommendations that few children were able to comply with, and if they were breastfed, they did not need solids to begin with.

Sadly all the experts seem to have made the same mistake: they recommended giving breastfed children the same foods that were necessary for artificially fed infants.

In the 1970s, formula had improved enough so that bottle-fed infants were no longer developing scurvy, rickets, or anaemia. Orange juice was no longer needed to avoid scurvy and the possible (more subtle) dangers of the early introduction of solids were starting to be observed: allergies, intolerances, and celiac disease. Little by little, solids were delayed, first to three months, then four, and now six. Personally I do not believe that the process has ended; it will be interesting to see what the future brings.

Epilogue
What if we were forced to eat?

The Charge of the Nutrition Brigade

The sun shone brightly in a cloudless sky, and the air carried the aroma of fresh-cut grass when Edmundo Tavares decided to go into The Goldfish, a pleasant, moderately priced restaurant. From his table, Edmundo had a lovely view of the park where the magnolias were in full bloom. An astute observer of human nature, he preferred however, to sit looking into the restaurant.

The clientele was as varied as they were fascinating. In front of him, an overweight and sweaty individual was eating greedily, stopping only to noisily gulp down incredible amounts of cheap wine. For a few seconds, Edmundo followed the movements of his double chin as if in a dream; the whitish mass undulated like dunes made of fine sand. It was not a scene that could entertain for very long and Edmundo soon ignored his corpulent neighbour to look at the wraithlike young woman who sat at the next table. "Wraithlike . . . what a poetic phrase," he said to himself. How many times had he read similar descriptions in a book? He associated "wraithlike" in his mind with a philosophic or religious manner, perhaps supernatural. Now, as he saw this pale girl, her eyes gazing away as if lost in thought sitting there in front of her untouched serving of pasta, he understood that "wraithlike" here had a much more earthly connotation, simply ethereal in terms of lacking substance, or you might say: "She's so thin, if she stands sideways she will disappear!"

In the centre of the room, next to the goldfish for which the establishment was named, sat several executives, properly attired (although the woman stood out because she was the only one not wearing a tie). They were passionately debating over a pile of documents and charts that covered both the food and the mobile phones on the table. Edmundo smiled, thinking about the tomato and grease-stained contracts. But wait, these were professionals; surely they were experts at reading a report over a bowl of salad without incident.

Farther back, in a discreet corner, a couple was gazing lovingly at each other, their hands entwined over the table. Nowadays, hands are entwined once again *over* the table! Funny how the world turns. Or perhaps his generation had few opportunities to entwine things in public places? "Am I growing old?" he thought, recalling with nostalgia other tables, other hands.

It was not easy to get lost for long in reminiscence, as the noisy laughter and talking from a group of students at the table behind him brought him quickly back to earth. He looked at them out of the corner of his eye. They joked merrily, totally unconcerned about social mores and unafraid to make fools of themselves. As it always happened when he looked at a group of young people, he thought he recognized a face. He quickly dismissed the idea as ridiculous; it could not be for they too would be forty years old by now.

His salad had just been brought out when a cold heavy silence descended upon the large room like waves in a pond. The feared black uniforms of the Nutritional Police (NP) were quickly lining up. He had not seen them come through the park; they must have come in the back door. There were half a dozen agents, under the command of a young, sharp-looking lieutenant. These officers, fresh out of the academy, were rigid and strict. Eager to justify their position, the new recruits were always the worst. Their own men were intimidated. They would not let anything go.

A middle-aged female agent quickly went up to the table where the executives sat. They had not had time to put away their contracts and reports. They were quickly confiscated. "No playing at the table!" The youngest executive tried to argue, but the woman stopped him with a glare. Resistance was pointless. Perhaps if they showed total submission and ate without complaining they would get their documents back after dessert.

All joking had come to a halt at the students' table. An arrest for bad eating behaviour could bring shame on their families and suspension from the university. They ate in absolute silence, sitting straight up in their seats, bringing the food to their mouths at a rhythmic pace. Were they perhaps sitting too straight, or eating too much in unison? Arms were lifted and lowered with choreographic precision. An observing agent seemed to have the vague sense that they were putting on a show, but no matter how carefully he looked he could not find anything illegal in their attitude so he opted to turn his back and disregard them. Several people at the surrounding tables were trying to hold back approving smiles: perhaps these young people were smarter than they seemed after all.

Screaming was heard from the kitchen. Every restaurant knew to get rid of any leftovers by washing them down the drain as soon as possible; but this time one of the kitchen helpers' inexperience had allowed the NP to discover a plate with half a ration of cannelloni. Laws outlawing leftover food on plates were unbendable. The owner stumbled over himself in explanations.

"We've always followed the rules, you know it. The client refused to finish his food and then ran off, we couldn't stop him. We have not had time to fill out the paperwork to denounce him; that is why we saved the plate. We needed a picture for the file . . . but we are clean, just look in the trash can, emp . . ."

With a dramatic gesture, the owner showed the trash container and words froze on his lips. Leftover stew! The new kitchen helper had made another mistake and this one could be fatal.

The sergeant stared at the owner, demanding an explanation. Before the others were able to speak, the kitchen helper stepped up, trembling: "I had to throw it away, I dropped a plate. But it did not break."

"We do not waste food," roared the owner. "Another mistake and you're fired."

Then, speaking respectfully to the sergeant: "He is new, it is getting harder and harder to find good help."

However, the shrewd way in which the kitchen worker had covered up his mistake was not lost on the owner. In those days, under constant threat of having your restaurant taken over by the Nutritional Police, quick thinking and sharp reflexes were important qualities.

Edmundo Tavares missed nothing of what was happening in the room, all the while seeming to give undivided attention to his salad. He congratulated himself on his choice: a light dish, one that strangely enough always seemed to have the approval of the NP. Nutritionals seemed delighted by green. The two lovebirds in the corner had stopped holding hands immediately, but they couldn't help giving each other loving looks once in a while. The agent who had been so severe with the executives seemed to relax her vigilance, but a cold stare from her lieutenant reminded her of her duties. She stood straight up and started to keep time with a shrill voice:

Eat in silence! Spoon to plate, spoon to mouth, one, two, spoon to plate, spoon to mouth, one, two!

The fat guy sitting in front of Edmundo was very nervous and was trying to catch glimpses of the officers. "He is trying to read their insignia," Edmundo understood suddenly. "He must be near-sighted."

The Nutritional SS (Super Stout) demanded weight above the mean, and the higher, the better; but they were in constant conflict with the Nutritional SA (Super Athletic) for whom the ideal weight was only between the 25th and 75th percentile. As a result of these internal battles of the regime, those individuals who had weights higher than the 75th percentile or between the 25th and 50th percentile had had a very difficult time. Not as hard, however, as those poor souls who were under the 25th percentile; the great majority of them had managed to go into exile before the borders were closed.

This time it was the Nutritional SS doing the inspection and the obese guy sighed in relief as soon as he was sure. He even dared to take an always risky step: "Waiter, the leg of lamb was delicious. Can I have seconds?"

The waiter's disgust was evident, but he had no choice. With the NP from the SS on the premises, seconds were guaranteed. The owner himself brought out the dish with a smile. Revenge, however, was sweet and subtle. The plate was piled high. The fat man paled when he saw it; he expected just a bit more, but this was way too much, even for him. Yet, to leave anything on a plate that he had asked for was one of the worst crimes.

Belatedly, the owner regretted his trick. The request for seconds, he understood, was not in order to take advantage of the situation, but only to seek protection. Hunted by the SA, the only safety for the obese was to have friends among the SS. Suddenly ashamed, he tried to offer him a way of escape:

"I'm sorry sir, we are out of custard," he stated cordially. "You will have to choose another dessert. May I suggest orange juice?"

"Certainly," responded the obese man, his eyes full of gratitude. Perhaps he would be able to finish the leg of lamb. He went right to it.

The lieutenant was standing by the fish tank. "Why is this fish not eating?"

"He just ate," defended the owner "but it doesn't matter." He pulled out some dry fish food and threw it in the tank. The goldfish hurried to devour it.

"Goldfish always have room for a little more food. That is why I chose them as the symbol for my establishment."

The lieutenant almost smiled. "It was a good idea to buy the goldfish," thought the owner, hoping that the incident at the trash can was forgotten. But the cold stare of the lieutenant was resolutely fixed on the thin girl. The silence became even more ominous. Not only did she seem to be under the 25th percentile (the stuffing in her bra could not hide her hollow cheeks), but her plate was still full of food and she was eating with excruciating slowness. Edmundo could tell that she was sweating, and he thought he heard her nervous heartbeat.

After watching her for a few painfully long seconds, the lieutenant gestured to one of the agents who resolutely approached the young lady.

Come on, eat a little. It's very good. There you go, that's great! You have to grow and get some meat on those bones. Come now, one more bite. There you go! You look so good when you eat. Are you tired honey? I'll help you. Give me your fork. Look, here's the plane, here it comes. Brrr, brrr! The plane with pasta for the girl. Good girl! Look, there's a birdie in the window! What a beautiful bird. See how he opens his beak? Good job, one more bite. Now this bite for grandma, this one for daddy. . . . Come on, let's not leave this yummy food. The cook made it with lots of love. You're almost finished. Don't you want to go to the movies today? Well, first you have to finish your food so you can be strong! Yummy! Look at the good girl; she's eating so well!

Slowly and painfully the pasta disappeared and the NP agent used a piece of bread to sop up the sauce and give it to the terrified woman to eat. There were still meat and potatoes to come! Edmundo, like many others in the restaurant, was holding his breath. It was plain she would never finish the second course.

The waiter brought out the meat. He had chosen the smallest cut and had only put a small serving of potatoes on the plate. He looked at the girl compassionately. She barely smiled in appreciation; the portion was still more than she would be able to eat and the waiter knew it. But he could not risk himself anymore; the NP sometimes made an owner weigh servings that looked suspiciously small.

The agent cut up the meat into small pieces and started again with her incessant prattle. Every spoonful was more painful than the last and the terror of one and irritation of the other became more and more evident. Edmundo, just like the other clients, tried to concentrate on his own plate, on the rhythmic back and forth of the fork. Trying not to look, not to think. Simply survive. How many times had Edmundo dreamed of being able to heroically stand up and proclaim with dignity: "Leave that young lady alone." Instead he swallowed his own cowardice as he overheard the police say to the woman: "See how that man eats? He is being so good! Come now, you've got to get big, like this man."

The young lady, with an empty gaze, opened and closed her mouth mechanically, while two tears slid down her cheeks.

"She has not swallowed in a while," thought Edmundo. Suddenly, with an unnerving sound, a mixture of a cough and nausea, the woman let a ball of dried up, chewed up meat fall from her mouth.

Lieutenant, she's refusing to swallow!

The official came closer with determined steps. A loud slap broke the silence. This is it, thought Edmundo, the end of planes and kind words. There was no pity for those who refused to swallow. He knew what would follow. They would make her eat that horrible repugnant ball of meat, and the rest of her food. They would force her mouth open, digging their iron fingers into her cheeks between her teeth so that if she tried to close her mouth she would bite herself. They would stuff her until she threw up, and then they would make her eat her own vomit. Edmundo closed his eyes, feeling totally miserable, and tried to take slow, deep breaths, to keep himself from vomiting while he listened to her desperate pleas:

I don't want any more! I don't want any more!

Edmundo forced his eyes open. All he saw was darkness. He understood suddenly that all had been a dream. "What a ridiculous dream," he thought. "Nutritional Police. Who could come up with such a thing?" However he still felt agitated and sweaty. It had all seemed so real. Especially that last plea.

I don't want any more! I don't want any more!

He was hearing the plea again! Terror made his spine tingle. But it was not a dream. It was his two-year-old daughter, Vanesa, who was crying out in her sleep in the next room. How strange, could we both have been having the same dream? No, she must be awake. That's it, I must have cried out in my sleep, and she is repeating it to get attention. The little devil! What kids will do to manipulate! The doctor warned us about this when he taught us how to get her to sleep. He said that she would try all sorts of things to get us to come to her room at night. I am not going, no sir! She has to learn to sleep alone and stop trying to get her own way.

By the way, one of these days we need to ask the doctor about the food thing. She eats less and less every day and now she's throwing up. We've got to do something with that child.

References

1. Illingworth, R. S., *The Normal Child. Some Problems of the Early Years and Their Treatment*, 10.ᵃ ed., Churchill Livingstone, Edinburgh, 1991.
2. Fomon, S. J., *Nutrition of Normal Infants*. Mosby Year Book, Inc., St. Louis 1992.
3. Van Den Boom, S. A. M., Kimber, A. C. and Morgan, J. B., Nutritional composition of home-prepared baby meals in Madrid. Comparison with commercial products in Spain and homemade meals in England, *Acta Pædiatrics*, 1997, 86: 57–62.
4. Butte, N. F., Wong, W. W., Hopkinson, J. M., Heinz, C. J., Mehta, N. R. y Smith, E. O. B., Energy requirements derived from total energy expenditure and energy deposition during the first 2 years of life, *Am. J. Clin. Nutr.*, 2000, 72: 1558–1569.
5. Dewey, K. G., Peerson, J. M. and Brown, K. H. et al., Growth of breastfed infants deviates from current reference data: a pooled analysis of US, Canadian, and European data sets, *Pediatrics*, 1995, 96: 495–503.
6. WHO, Working Group on Infant Growth. *An evaluation of infant growth*, Document WHO/NUT/94.8, OMS, Geneva, 1994.
7. Dewey, K. G., Growth patterns of breastfed infants and the current status of growth charts for infants, *J. Hum. Lact.*, 1998,14: 89–92.
8. Von Kries, R., Koletzko, B., Sauerwald, T., Von Mutius, E., Barnert, D., Grunert, V. and Von Voss, H., Breast feeding and obesity: cross sectional study, *BMJ*, 1999, 319: 147–150.
9. Grummer-Strawn, L. M. and Mei, Z., Centers for Disease Control and Prevention Pediatric Nutrition Surveillance System. Does breast-feeding protect against pediatric overweight? Analysis of longitudinal data from the Centers for Disease Control and Prevention Pediatric Nutrition Surveillance System, *Pediatrics*, 2004, 113: 81–86.
10. Räihä, N. C. R. and Axelsson, I. E., Protein nutrition during infancy. An update, *Pediatr. Clin. N. Amer.*, 1995, 42: 745–764.
11. Howie, P. W., Houston, M. J., Cook, A. et al., How long should a breast feed last?, *Early Hum. Dev.*, 1981, 5: 71–77.
12. Woolridge, M. W., Baby-controlled breastfeeding: Biocultural implications, in Stuart-Macadam, P. and Dettwyler, K. A., *Breastfeeding, Biocultural Perspectives*, Aldine de Gruyter, New York, 1995.
13. Woolridge, M. W., Ingram, J. C. and Baum, J. D., Do changes in pattern of breast usage alter the baby's nutrient intake?, *Lancet*, 1990, 336: 395-397.
14. Birch, L. L. and Fisher, J. A., Appetite and eating behaviour in children, *Pediatr. Clin. N. Amer.*, 1995, 42: 931–953.
15. Birch, L. L., Johnson, S. L., Andresen, G. et al., The variability of young children's energy intake, *N. Eng. J. Med.*, 1991, 324: 232–235.
16. Shea, S., Stein, A. D., Basch, C. E. et al., Variability and self-regulation of

energy intake in young children in their everyday environment, *Pediatrics*, 1992, 90: 542–546.

17. Fisher, J. O. and Birch, L. L., Restricting access to palatable foods affects children's behavioral response, food selection, and intake, *Am. J. Clin. Nutr.*, 1999, 69: 1264–1272.

18. ESPGAN, Committee on Nutrition, Guidelines on infant nutrition. III. Recommendations for infant feeding, *Acta Pædiatr. Scand.*, 1982, suppl. 302.

19. Complementary feeding: A commentary by the ESPGHAN Committee on Nutrition, *J. Pediatr. Gastroenterol. Nutr.,* 2008; 46:99–110.

20. American Academy of Pediatrics Committee on Nutrition, On the feeding of supplemental foods to infants, *Pediatrics*, 1980, 65: 1178–1181.

21. American Academy of Pediatrics Section on Breastfeeding, Breast-feeding and the use of human milk, *Pediatrics*, 2005, 115: 496–506. http://aappolicy. aappublications.org/cgi reprint/pediatrics; 115/2/496.pdf

22. American Academy of Pediatrics Work Group on Breastfeeding, Breast-feeding and the use of human milk, *Pediatrics*, 1997, 100: 1035–1039.

23. UNICEF, WHO, UNESCO, UNFPA, UNDP, UNAIDS, WFP and the World Bank, Facts for Life., 3rd ed, 2002. http://www.unicef.org/publications/index_4387.html

24. Cohen, R. J., Brown, K. H., Canahuati, J. et al., Effects of age of introduction of complementary foods on infant breast milk intake, total energy intake, and growth: a randomised intervention study in Honduras, *Lancet*, 1994, 343: 288–293.

25. Klaus, M. H., The frequency of suckling. A neglected but essential ingredient of breast-feeding, *Obstet. Gynecol. Clin. N. Amer.*, 1987, 14: 623–633.

26. Daly, S. E. J. and Hartmann, P. E., Infant demand and milk supply. Part 2: The short-term control of milk synthesis in lactating women, *J. Hum. Lact.*, 1995, 11: 27–37.

27. Weile, B., Cavell, B., Nivenius, K. y Krasilnikoff, P. A., Striking differences in the incidence of childhood celiac disease between Denmark and Sweden: a plausible explanation, *J. Pediatr. Gastroenterol. Nutr.*, July 1995, 21: 64–68.

28. Ivarsson, A., Hernell, O., Stenlund, H. and Persson L. A., Breast-feeding protects against celiac disease, *Am. J. Clin. Nutr.*, 2002, 75: 914–921.

29. Complementary feeding: A commentary by the ESPGHAN Committee on Nutrition, *J. Pediatr. Gastroenterol. Nutr.*, 2008.

30. American Academy of Pediatrics, Committee on Nutrition. Hypoallergenic infant formulas, *Pediatrics*, 2000;106:346–349.

31. Complementary feeding: A commentary by the ESPGHAN Committee on Nutrition, *J. Pediatr. Gastroenterol. Nutr.*, 2008.

32. Greer F. R., Sicherer S. H., Burks A. W., American Academy of Pediatrics Committee on Nutrition; American Academy of Pediatrics Section on Allergy and Immunology. Effects of early nutritional interventions on the development of atopic disease in infants and children: the role of maternal

dietary restriction, breastfeeding, timing of introduction of complementary foods, and hydrolyzed formulas, *Pediatrics*, 2008; 121:183–191.

33. Macknin, M. L., Medendorp, S. V. and Maier, M. C., Infant sleep and bedtime cereal, *Am. J. Dis. Child.*, 1989, 143: 1066–1068.
34. Comité de Lactancia Materna de la AEP. Recomendaciones para la lactancia materna, 2008. http://www.aeped.es/pdfdocs/ lacmat.pdf
35. Fernández Núñez, J. M., Sendín González, C., Herrera, P. et al., «Doctor, el niño no me come», como demanda de consulta, Atención Primaria, 1997, 20: 554–556.
36. Comité de Nutrición de la Asociación Española de Pediatría, Indicaciones de las fórmulas antirregurgitación, *An. Esp. Pediatr.*, 2000, 52: 369–371.
37. American Academy of Pediatrics, Committee on Nutrition, The use and misuse of fruit juice in pediatrics, *Pediatrics*, 2001, 107: 1210–1213.
38. Sanders, T. A. B., Vegetarians diets and children, *Pediatr. Clin. N. Amer.*, 1995, 42: 955–965.
39. Norris, J., Vitamin B_{12} Recommendations for Vegans, http://www.veganoutreach.org/health/b12rec.html
40. Hood, S., The vegan diet for infants and children. http://www.scienzavegetariana.it/rubriche/cong2002/vegcon_infant_diet_en.html
41. Bowlby, J., *The Making and Breaking of Affectional Bonds*, Routledge, London, 2000.
42. Dewey, K. G. and Brown, K. H., Update on technical issues concerning complementary feeding of young children in developing countries and implications for intervention programs, *Food. Nut. Bull.*, 2003, 24: 2–28.
43. Ulecia and Cardona, R., *Arte de criar a los niños*, 2.ª ed., Administración de la Revista de Medicina y Cirugía Prácticas, Madrid, 1906.
44. Puig y Roig, P., *Puericultura o arte de criar bien a los hijos*, Librería Subirana, Barcelona, 1927.
45. Goday, S., *Alimentació del nen durant la primera infància*, Monografies Mèdiques, 19, Barcelona, 1928.
46. Roig i Raventós, J., *Nocions de puericultura*, 4.ª ed., Políglota, Barcelona, 1932.
47. Roig i Raventós, J., *Nocions de puericultura*, 5.ª ed., Políglota, Barcelona, 1936.
48. Roig i Raventós, J., *Nocions de puericultura*, 7.ª ed., Políglota, Barcelona, 1947.
49. Ramos, R., *Puericultura. Higiene, educación y alimentación en la primera infancia, tomo I*, Barcelona, 1941.
50. Blancafort, M., *Puericultura actual*, Bruguera, Barcelona, 1979.
51. Muñoz, J., *Madre... cría a tu hijo!*, Barcelona, 1941.

Index

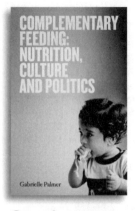
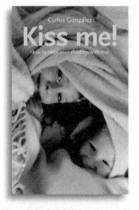
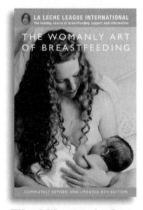
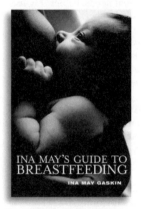